Dedication

*This book is dedicated to
The True Self wherein lies
happiness and contentment*

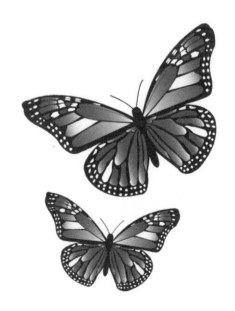

Help for Depression and Anxiety

How to have a Happy and Healthy Nervous System

Dr Sandra Cabot

Help for Depression and Anxiety
Copyright © 2009 Dr Sandra Cabot

First Published 2009 by WHAS Pty Ltd

WHAS Pty Ltd – Australia
P. O. Box 689, Camden NSW, 2570 Australia
Phone 02 4655 8855

SCB Inc. – United States of America
PO Box 5070 Glendale AZ USA 85312
Phone 623 334 3232

www.weightcontroldoctor.com.au
www.cabothealth.com.au

ISBN 0–9757437–2–4

1) Mental Health 2) Depression 3) Anxiety 4) Panic Attacks 5) Post Natal Depression 6) Nervous System 7) Happiness

Author biography

Dr Sandra McRae Cabot MBBS, DRCOG is the Medical and Executive Director of the Australian National Health Advisory Service. She graduated with honours in Medicine and Surgery from the University of Adelaide in South Australia in 1975.

Dr Cabot began her medical career in 1980 as a GP Obstetrician-Gynaecologist and practised in Sydney Australia. During the mid 1980s she spent 6 months working as a volunteer doctor at the Leyman hospital, which was the largest missionary hospital in Northern India.

Dr Cabot is an experienced commercial pilot and flies herself to seminars throughout Australia, often visiting remote areas. Dr Cabot and her Beechcraft Baron aircraft do regular work for the Angel Flight Charity, which provides free transport for patients with chronic and severe disabilities in remote Australian areas.

Dr Cabot has conducted health seminars all over the world and is frequently asked to lecture for numerous health organisations such as The American Liver Foundation and the Annual Hepatitis Symposium.

Dr Cabot still has an active medical practice and does research into liver diseases.

Dr Cabot believes that the most important health issues for people today are-

- The control of obesity and the prevention of diabetes
- Educating our children about self esteem, good diet and healthy lifestyle
- Making hormone replacement therapy safe and as natural as possible
- The use of specific nutritional supplements to treat and prevent diseases
- Educating doctors and naturopaths so that they can work together using evidence based holistic medicine to achieve the

best outcomes for patients
- The effective treatment of mental and emotional illness
- A supportive and well educated community where people have the confidence and knowledge to find the best health care

Dr Cabot has written several ground breaking books –

Don't Let Your Hormones Ruin Your Life

Hormone Replacement – The Real Truth – Balance your hormones naturally and swing from the chandeliers!

The Body Shaping Diet

The Liver Cleansing Diet

The Healthy Liver and Bowel Book

Boost Your Energy

Raw Juices can save your Life

Can't lose weight? – You could have Syndrome X

Cholesterol - The Real Truth

The Ultimate Detox Diet

Tired of not sleeping? A holistic guide to a good night's sleep

Alzheimer's – what you must know to protect your brain

The Dr Sandra Cabot Recipe Collection

Bird Flu – Your Personal Survival Guide

Your Thyroid Problems Solved

Diabetes type 2 – you can reverse it naturally

Low carb cocktail party – recipes for low carb drinks and food

Want to lose weight... but hooked on food?

The Breast Cancer Prevention Guide

Magnesium the Miracle Mineral

www.sandracabot.com

Contents

Introduction

Depression – how to get help and recover

Incidence of depression

Depression has recently been quoted in the newspapers as "the most predicted common ailment of the 21st century". Depression is still mostly misunderstood and unfortunately the stigma associated with it remains pervasive. This is because a depressive illness often masquerades as something else, and it is still minimised as an illness; however it can wreak havoc in the quality of a person's physical and mental health.

Undiagnosed depression exacts an enormous toll in people's lives and the cost of undiagnosed depression has ballooned to as much as 5 billion dollars a year. These losses come from low productivity, employee absenteeism, serious accidents, marital break-up and suicide. Perhaps the greatest cost of depression is in lost time, because for depressed individuals the days pass without meaning or enjoyment.

Every year nearly 60,000 Australians attempt suicide. The World Health Organisation predicts that by the year 2020, five of the ten leading medical problems worldwide will be stress related.

Many people with depression do not seek effective help and suffer needlessly. Depression has been described under various terms from heart-break, dejection, the blues, and involutional melancholia. Today psychiatrists have called it clinical depression.

We need a holistic approach

To achieve good and lasting results in overcoming emotional illness (incorporating depression and anxiety) we need to address all possible causal factors. This can be difficult because there is a shortage of medical doctors and psychiatrists in Australia and emotional problems are often associated with financial problems, so people try to help themselves and battle on. Many feel dispirited or ashamed and give up trying to get help especially if their emotional problems recur.

The worse things you can do are not to seek help or self medicate with alcohol or other drugs. If you do these things you will gradually deteriorate over time.

Thankfully today there are some excellent resources on the Internet and I have listed these helpful websites, along with some good self help books on pages 117-128.

The holistic approach to emotional distress and imbalance addresses the following issues –

- Counselling from a good doctor, psychologist or a professional counsellor – this can often be arranged through your local doctor (GP) who can set up a care plan for you
- Nutritional deficiencies and the need for supplements
- Poor diet and lifestyle
- Relaxation techniques
- Support groups
- Hormonal causes of emotional distress and mental fatigue
- Genetic factors causing inherited depression and anxiety
- The need for specific prescribed medication tailor made for the individual

Holistic treatment means that lasting recovery from emotional illness is within everyone's reach.

There are a few important points to consider:

- Your treatment does not have to be expensive and indeed it is wise to be wary of treatments or courses that cost exorbitant amounts because they may not be sustainable.

- You need to be wary of fanatical approaches towards the treatment of emotional illness. For example there are some religions and some programs (often found on the Internet) that are totally antagonistic towards antidepressant drugs or indeed any form of pharmacological drugs that can be prescribed for emotional and/or mental illness. The proponents of this negative approach to modern day drugs, and the pharmaceutical companies that manufacture them, are misguided by brain washing and fanaticism. Such people really do not have the professional expertise or clinical experience to back up their concepts.

In this book I aim to give you practical help and understanding of the use of prescribed antidepressant drugs, natural hormones and natural dietary supplements that can strengthen the emotional system and indeed your whole brain. I think that there is a lack of awareness in the general community about the use of antidepressant drugs and they are frequently misunderstood. Many doctors are unfortunately unaware of the use of natural hormones such as progesterone, which can be a wonderful regulator of disturbed emotions in women.

In this book I give you a list of brain boosting foods to optimise the physical and functional integrity of your brain.

Only by addressing all these factors can we achieve the best possible outcome for every individual who suffers with some form of emotional distress.

In this book I provide a holistic approach to overcoming emotional distress and I have outlined a plan that you can follow to address all the factors that may be overloading your nervous system.

Chapter One

Why do we become vulnerable to depression?

Causes of emotional illness

1. Genetic factors can make us prone to emotional illness and it is important to look at your family history. Researchers have discovered specific physical characteristics in our genes that will make us prone to depression, obsessive compulsive disorders and anxiety, and these often manifest at an early age. Knowing your genetic weaknesses can help you to be better prepared for everyday stresses and to arrange your life so that pressure does not build up to intolerable levels. Australian researchers say that more than a fifth of the population have a genetic predisposition to major depression triggered by a string of stressful life events. The study, published in the *British Journal of Psychiatry*, found that a gene that controls the neurotransmitter serotonin is crucial. The researchers found that people with a short version of the serotonin-transporter gene have an 80 per cent chance of developing clinical depression if they have three or more negative life events in a year. In contrast people with a long or more protective version of the gene only have a 30 per cent risk of becoming depressed under similar circumstances.

2. Personality Types are important and some studies indicate that people with pessimistic thinking, low self esteem and little sense of control and who are prone to excess worry are more likely to become depressed. Some psychologists have argued that women have been raised to be like this, and that is why they develop depression at a higher rate than men do. They say that women are generally more passive and dependent and less able to express anger because they have been raised to think it is an unacceptable emotion. However when anger is denied and turned inward, depression is often the result.

3. The past and present environment has a big influence on the emotional state. People with a history of childhood sexual abuse are more likely to become depressed in adulthood. Psychologists have found that exposure to abuse may lead to a higher incidence of depression, due to feelings of low self worth, self blame, a sense of helplessness and social isolation. Poverty causes stresses of uncertainty, isolation and poor access to resources, which can lead to sadness.

4. The loss or non-achievement of something in your life that is important to your self-esteem. This could be the loss of a relationship, a high paying job, loss of status, financial loss, the loss of health, the loss of youth, and the loss of virility. These losses can leave a gaping hole in one's ego, which can be difficult to replace with positive thoughts alone. Loss often leads to stress, which then leads to anxiety, and then after several weeks or months depression sets in.

5. The sense of not being in control of one's destiny can lead to stress and frustration. Globally there is a trend towards large organisations and corporations and the direction of employees is often exerted by remote electronic control. Decisions are focused on pleasing directors, top executives and shareholders and corporations do not appreciate the huge emotional and financial toll that depression in their employees will have. Challenging pressures in the work place can be very energising if they occur in an atmosphere of high morale. We have lost the personal touch in a corporate world that is valued in dollar numbers only.

6. Hormonal imbalances can lead to depression and anxiety and the most common ones are lack of progesterone in women and lack of testosterone in men. Premenstrual depression can often be alleviated with a combination of natural progesterone cream and nutritional supplements. Depression during the peri-menopausal years can often be dramatically improved by fine-tuning the body with a combination of bio-identical hormones such as natural oestrogen, progesterone, DHEA (dehydroepiandrosterone) and testosterone. For more details see my book called "*HRT – The Real Truth – Balance your hormones and swing from the chandeliers!*" Depression after childbirth or a miscarriage is a serious and relatively common illness that often lingers for years without adequate treatment. Postnatal depression can respond

very quickly to antidepressant drugs, nutritional supplements and natural progesterone cream.

7. Lifestyle and diet play an important role and people who abuse drugs and/or alcohol have higher rates of depression. Alcohol, many recreational drugs, and some prescription medications can lead to depression. Those with poor diets and poor lifestyle habits are more likely to suffer with mood disorders.

8. Nutritional deficiencies of omega 3 essential fatty acids, vitamin D, antioxidants, minerals and some amino acids can lead to chemical imbalances in the brain which can lead to emotional illness and cognitive decline. Deficiencies of folic acid and vitamin B6 can predispose an individual to depression, and cause that individual to not respond to antidepressant medication.

9. Inflammation can promote depression. Inflammation occurs when the body's immune cells (or fat cells) produce chemicals referred to as cytokines. Inflammation occurs as a response to an infection, allergy, autoimmune condition, chronic pain, obesity, diabetes and several other factors. The cytokines produced impair the ability of serotonin to function. Therefore, each of the conditions listed above increase the risk of an individual suffering with depression. Inflammation can also be one factor responsible for an individual not responding to antidepressant medication.

No matter what the cause of our depression is, it is true that the most stressful thing in life is often between our ears. It is in the mind that threats and emptiness are perceived. The greatest battlefield of life is usually in our own mind and when we can no longer fight alone for victory, thankfully we can turn towards modern day psychiatry and holistic medicine. To me the definition of holistic medicine is healing that helps the mind, body and spirit.

Why should depression be treated early?

There are many reasons that a depressive illness should be treated. In this modern age, depression can be treated successfully and it's sad to see someone suffer unnecessarily, especially for a long time.

New studies reported in the October 2008 edition of the journal *The Archives of General Psychiatry* have found that chronic major depression may result in loss of grey matter in important parts of the brain. This is an important reason that the treatment of depression should not be delayed, as the adverse changes in the physical structure of the brain caused by untreated depression, may make the depression worse; thus it becomes a self perpetuating illness. Researchers from the University of Munich, Germany, performed MRI scans of the brains of 38 inpatients with major depression and compared them to MRI scans in healthy control patients at 3 year intervals. Over a 3 year period the researchers discovered that the grey matter shrunk in important areas of the brain concerned with intellect, character, judgement, emotions and memory in the 38 depressed subjects. In contrast, this did not happen to a significant degree in the healthy non depressed control patients.

The researchers concluded that during depressive episodes grey matter density shrinks in the emotional and intellectual areas of the brain – namely the limbic and frontal cortex. The more severe the depression was, the more severe the physical changes in the brain became. The researchers could not be sure why the depression caused these important areas of the brain to physically deteriorate.

These findings necessitate the need for further research and also stimulate us to hypothesize. I am sure that many of these adverse physical changes in the brain could be prevented if not only early treatment of a depressive illness was initiated, but just as importantly, a holistic approach to treatment was embraced. The brain is a "plastic organ" and the physical structures of the brain can be improved with appropriate nutritional supplements and diet, as well as antidepressant drugs if needed. Cognitive therapies and the stimulation of new learning and interaction can also cause the brain tissue to grow and form new neural pathways or circuits. The brain is like a muscle – if you don't use it, it will atrophy.

Chapter Two

How do you know if you have an emotional illness?

Symptoms of depression

These can vary a lot between individuals and depression often exists for years without correct diagnosis and treatment being made. This is because depression can masquerade as many different illnesses.

Symptoms of depression may include the following:

Persistently depressed or unhappy moods, overwhelming feelings of sadness, doom and gloom

Irritability and grumpiness

Loss of interest

Loss of pleasure in all usual activities and hobbies

Loss of motivation

Withdrawing from friends and social activity

An increased use of drugs, alcohol or smoking to cope

Changes in appetite leading to weight gain or weight loss

Bowel disturbances such as irritable bowel syndrome

Changes in sleep, often associated with early morning awakening and not being able to get back to sleep

Mental and/or physical agitation

Mental and/or physical slowness

Impaired concentration and memory

Suicidal thoughts or thoughts of harming yourself

Feelings of pessimism and hopelessness

Loss of interest in sex and/or impotence

Increased fatigue

Inappropriate feelings of guilt or obligation

Inappropriate feelings of worthlessness

Low self esteem

Loss of assertiveness

Loss of emotional resilience

Feeling emotionally numb

Feeling too serious

Worrying excessively about physical health, money or the future

Difficulty making decisions

Loss of confidence

Reduced ability to take normal and/or natural risks

Thinking excessively about the past (rumination)

Feelings of excessive resentment

Being unusually self-critical

Increased headaches

Increased general aches and pains in the muscles and bones (fibromyalgia)

A feeling of heaviness in the centre of the chest (can be compared to a heavy heart)

A feeling of weight on the shoulders

Increased sighing

Symptoms of anxiety

Breathlessness

Muscle or whole body tremor

Muscle pains or cramps due to continual muscle tension

Heaviness of the limbs

Racing or pounding heart beat

Missing or thudding heart beat (palpitations)

Increased blood pressure

Increased sweating

Dizziness

Light headedness

Feelings of unreality and loss of definition of the self – patients often say things like "I feel weird, I feel unreal, I am not myself, I feel like I am in a bad dream"

Reduced ability to take normal and/or natural risks

An increased use of drugs, alcohol or smoking to cope

Bowel disturbances such as irritable bowel syndrome

Indigestion and/or reflux

Changes in sleep, often associated with difficulty falling asleep and broken sleep

Panic attacks which produce a feeling of total loss of control and impending disaster

Mental and/or physical agitation

Feeling anxious and tense

A feeling of weight on the shoulders

Fear of places such as: claustrophobia (fear of confined spaces) or agoraphobia (fear of leaving home or a secure place)

Asthma

Headaches

Decreased libido or impotence

Anxiety can be triggered by or aggravated by the following factors:

- Hypoglycaemia
- Hyperthyroidism (over active thyroid) or hypothyroidism (under active thyroid)
- Hormonal imbalances such as during menopause or PMS
- Nutritional deficiencies – particularly of magnesium, choline and vitamins B1, B3 and B5.
- Excessive consumption of stimulants, such as sugar, caffeine or nicotine
- Consumption of artificial sweeteners, particularly aspartame (food additive 951).
- Heavy alcohol consumption
- A sedentary lifestyle with very little exercise.

You will see that depression and anxiety share many common symptoms and indeed the two illnesses often overlap. With depression the feelings of sadness and hopelessness are predominant whereas in anxiety states the feelings of loss of control and panic are predominant. In most cases of prolonged anxiety some degree of depression will eventually set in.

The horrible physical symptoms of anxiety can make the patient much more anxious and so we have a snowball effect with increasing symptoms causing more anxiety which causes worsening symptoms. For example it can be extremely frightening and disabling to feel your heart racing, a heavy pressure in the chest and shortness of breath – you feel as though you are about to have a heart attack or die. The reality of such an anxiety attack is that you do not have a heart or lung problem, you have a chemical imbalance caused by the flooding of your body with adrenalin. Once your body breaks the adrenalin down you will return to normal and what a relief that will be!

Anxious patients can have many different symptoms and thus may consult various specialists – such as a heart specialist, a chest physician, a gastroenterologist or a neurologist, and yet after tests are done the doctors cannot find a physical cause for their horrible symptoms. The symptoms can be treated with drugs such as antacids, sleeping tablets, muscle relaxants, pain killers, anti-spasm medications, muscle relaxants etc; however if the cause, namely the anxiety, is not treated, new and recurring symptoms may occur. What a horrible state of mental and physical health to be stuck in for the rest of your life. Thankfully by providing understanding and treatment of the cause of the symptoms, namely anxiety, we do not have to lead a life of suffering.

Psychotic depression

This is characterised by delusions of various types and is more common in the elderly and the malnourished. There may be delusions of poverty or guilt, which cause them to live in squalor, isolation and deprivation. The sufferer may believe that their body is invaded by evil spirits or that parts of their body have rotted away. These patients often refuse treatment because they are confused and mistrustful. They require hospitalisation and specialised treatment which is life saving.

Obsessive Compulsive Disorders (OCD) associated with depression

Some forms of depression may be associated with obsessive compulsive thoughts and behaviour such as over checking things, counting things, repetitive hand washing or obsessive thoughts of germs and filth. The sufferer may think they are vulnerable to diseases or evil spirits and may have to perform repetitive rituals to ward these dangers off. These fears and anxieties may become chronic and cause wasted time, distraction, depression and inability to function.

Anorexia nervosa is a type of obsessive compulsive depression where the patient develops a morbid fear of fat or weight gain. The patient becomes obsessed with not eating so they can lose all their body fat. Their perception is distorted and they see themselves as ugly and fat when in reality they look painfully thin.

Obsessive compulsive disorders associated with depression often respond extremely well to antidepressant drugs and cognitive behavioural therapy. If strong delusions persist, other types of medications may need to be added to the antidepressants.

Bipolar Mood Disorder (also known as manic depression)

Around 1 in 20 people will suffer with a bipolar mood disorder. When a person presents with a first episode of depression there is a 20% chance that it will progress to a bipolar disorder. In this type of illness, depression alternates with periods of manic behaviour. During the manic episode the patient becomes hyperactive and loses the ability to think rationally. During periods of mania the patient often feels very well with high energy levels, elevated mood and delusions of grandeur. They may spend huge amounts of money and believe they have super human powers. Their increased physical and mental energy often prevents them from sleeping for days at a time. They may think they are able to achieve great things and get themselves into difficult situations.

In summary, signs of mania typically include

    Racing thoughts and pressured speech

    Distractibility

    Mental and physical agitation

    Participation in high risk activities such as – alcohol and drug abuse, risky business ventures, sexual liaisons, gambling, shopping sprees

Increased sex drive

Insomnia and loss of need to sleep

Enormous energy levels

Excess self esteem and confidence

Excess socialisation – constant phone calls all night, wild parties, annoying friends or relatives with visits and bursts of creativity

When the manic episode ends it is replaced with severe depression.

It is important to differentiate simple depression from bipolar disorder because if the depressive phase of the bipolar disorder is treated with antidepressant drugs alone, bipolar depression is likely to develop into mania or rapid cycling of moods from very low moods to very high moods. Antidepressant drugs alone should not be used to treat bipolar illness.

The risk of suicide is quite high in bipolar disorder, especially during the depressive phase which is difficult to treat, and for this reason timely referral to a specialist psychiatrist is essential. Electroconvulsive therapy may be needed and is very effective for severe depression in bipolar illness and may often prevent suicide.

Manic depression is often inherited and may be triggered by the excessive use of alcohol or recreational drugs. This illness is more severe than regular or simple depression and different drugs such as mood stabiliser drugs are required to control the symptoms. Mood stabilising drugs include lithium, olanzapine, quetiapine and lamotrigine. It may be necessary to add an anti-convulsant drug (such as valproate) to one of these mood stabilisers and the combination of lithium and valproate is usually well tolerated by patients.

If mood stabilising drugs alone have not been effective in alleviating the depression, most doctors will add a SSRI antidepressant drug to the patient's drug regime. Lamotrigine can work well as an antidepressant and a mood stabiliser and is generally well tolerated by the patient. Lamotrigine is somewhat expensive and can cause a severe immune type reaction known as "Stevens-Johnson Syndrome". Often the time proven and oldest drug in the stable, lithium, works the best of all for long term control of bipolar illness.

People who have suffered with manic depression should avoid alcohol and drugs and usually need to stay on long term medication. Supportive counselling and psychotherapy are also essential.

The natural therapies discussed in this book will help those with bipolar to stay mentally and physically healthier and may prevent relapses or reduce the severity of their relapses.

Risk of suicide

The presence of suicidal thoughts or plans must be taken very seriously and these should be asked about. There is no evidence that broaching the subject of suicidal thoughts in a depressed patient is dangerous – in other words it has not been shown to increase the risk of suicide occurring. Indeed many depressed patients have these thoughts and are often relieved to be able to talk about suicidal thoughts in an open manner as they may feel too guilty to be able to talk about it.

The following factors increase the risk of suicide

Male sex
Older age group
Adolescent age group
Unemployment
Isolation – being divorced, separated or socially alone
Chronic medical illness or pain
Drug or alcohol abuse
Access to firearms
A past history of suicide attempts
Making active plans for suicide
Making final plans – organising a will, saying goodbyes

It can be difficult to broach the subject of suicide with a depressed patient, so here are some suggested strategic questions you could ask:

Do you ever wish you would not wake up in the morning?

Are things so bad you think it is not worth living?

Do you think your family would be better off without you?

Have you ever thought of harming yourself or trying to end your life?

Have you made any plans to end your life?

Self esteem

I find the topic of self esteem a fascinating one as it affects our life's potential in such a profound way. Self esteem is based on the way you see yourself and the value you put on yourself and in reality can be such a fragile thing. I have found that self esteem in many wonderful people I know can be very low, although this is not always obvious.

In this modern superficial world many people have been educated to base their self esteem on material things such as

- How successful you are in your career
- How much money you make
- How prestigious your work is
- How you look
- Your body weight
- If you have full time and well paid employment
- How many friends you have
- How many assets you have
- How young you are
- How society and your circle of friends view you

Self esteem is often incorrectly measured against the stereotypes of modern society. For example a beautiful woman is portrayed in the media as incredibly slim and perfect and able to afford fashionable clothes. This gives many young women an impossible standard to which they must aspire to feel attractive and therefore valued. No wonder we have such a high incidence of eating disorders in young women. The condition of self loathing and hating one's own body and/or appearance is called "dysmorphophobia" and the desire to change one's appearance becomes an unhealthy obsession. These people often have repeated plastic surgery with a poor outcome. The media could do a lot to help overcome the stereotype of beauty and success by using more actors and models of different shapes, sizes and ages. Our society is very ageist and does not place enough value on the experiences and ability of older people.

Paradoxically self esteem problems are more common in young people who are in the physical and mental prime of their lives. Such young people often turn to alcohol or drugs to overcome their low self esteem and present a brave front to the world. The incidence of teenage suicide is very high and the fact that these young people feel worthless and misplaced is something we need to work on in the family home, schools and the community. Many problems originate in childhood where our self image and self value is shaped. Parents and teachers need to become more sensitive to the children they have and educate, so that self esteem problems can be picked up early on before they become ingrained. Many children need to be given positive encouragement and feedback on a continual basis, encouraging their expression and concerns. If a child develops behavioral problems or inexplicable physical symptoms such as poor sleep, abdominal pain, hair pulling, muscular ticks, facial grimaces etc, these are often signs of hidden anxiety, depression or nutritional deficiencies of magnesium, B vitamins or omega three fatty acids. Children need to be told positive things about themselves, and their unique personality and traits can be encouraged. Broken families, abandonment and sexual abuse issues are situations where self esteem may be damaged if special attention and early intervention does not take place.

Interestingly I have observed that it is often the nicest people who suffer with low self esteem. This may be associated with depression and anxiety and feelings of guilt and excessive obligation. They may incorrectly believe that they are responsible for the problems of other people in their family or circle of friends. Conversely most psychopaths or mass murderers such as Hitler, Stalin and Pol Pot had huge egos and never felt any guilt for the suffering they caused.

True self esteem is not based upon how you think others see you; rather it is based upon the value you put on yourself as a human being. I only learnt this once I became a popular author. I was surprised, even shocked, by the criticism I received from several of my colleagues about the subjects of my first few books. Initially I felt intimidated about this and questioned myself as to what was wrong with my books. I believed that I was trying to help people with the knowledge I had gained by excellent training and extensive research into my chosen health subjects. Some of the criticism I received bordered on defamation and was trying to injure my credibility, so much so that I thought to myself that perhaps I should stop writing and promoting my holistic theories on health. However my readers thought differently! – they enjoyed my books and I received thousands of letters and emails of congratulations, thanks and pleas for help. So I persisted and indeed I don't think I could have stopped, as I have always been a writer even as a child. Eventually I wrote a famous book called *The Liver Cleansing Diet* which sold over 2 million copies worldwide and was translated into 6 languages. One critic of this book became very upset with me and even tried to have me deregistered from the medical profession! This was a little scary and unsettling and initially I did not know how to handle it. But I persisted, as I had enough self esteem to trust and believe in myself. I knew that my research and clinical experience were valuable and that my readers appreciated my help.

These experiences taught me several things – one of these was that you can and should believe in yourself even when others don't; the other was the power of reverse psychology. The more negative things the detractor of my Liver Cleansing Diet book kept saying, the more well known the book became – it became controversial and thus more interesting to the general public. Thus the book sold more and more and won the People's Choice Award for the most popular non fiction book of 1997. I could not have hired a better PR agent than my detractor, whose efforts got me onto prime time television and radio and into leading newspapers.

Life will work its magic if you let go of fear and live your life as an exclamation and not as an explanation.

Chapter Three

Brain chemistry –
the chemistry of happiness

The brain can be compared to a battery – when it is fully charged our emotions are normal, pleasurable and stable. If the brain becomes "flat" it will act like a flat battery and we will feel flat, fatigued, and emotionally unstable. We know that for a battery in our car to work properly it must be fully charged and the electrical charge of a battery is maintained by the correct combination of chemicals in the battery. Similarly the electrical energy or "charge" in our brain is maintained by the correct amount and balance of chemicals in the brain. These brain chemicals are made by our brain cells and the most important ones are serotonin, noradrenalin and dopamine. These brain chemicals are known as neurotransmitters. If these neurotransmitters become depleted or excessive, the electrical activity of the brain will become dysfunctional. This can result in depression and/or anxiety.

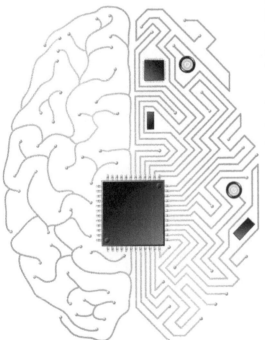

I find this analogy of the brain to a battery is helpful for my patients and they can then relate to their symptoms as being due to a chemical imbalance and not just an attitude or psychological problem.

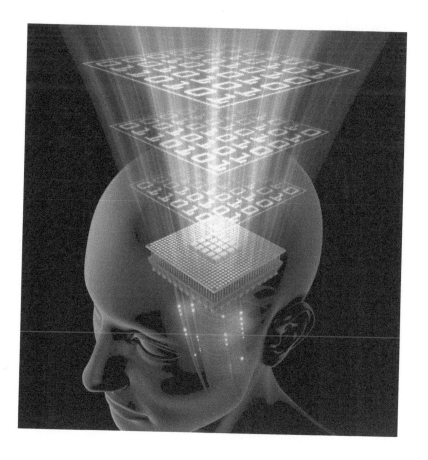

Serotonin – the happy chemical!

When it comes to our moods and the way that we generally enjoy the pleasures of life, serotonin is a very important brain chemical.

Serotonin is a remarkable brain messenger and adequate amounts of serotonin are required for

- Stable moods
- Feelings of happiness and contentment
- Proper and restful sleep
- A healthy libido
- Prevention of premenstrual syndrome
- Prevention of headaches
- Control of anxiety

Depressive illness is often caused by or associated with abnormally low levels of serotonin in the brain. Most antidepressant drugs increase the amounts of serotonin available to the brain cells.

Symptoms of serotonin deficiency

The following are all possible symptoms of serotonin deficiency:

Bad temper and aggression

Irritability

Insomnia

Depression

Eating disorders

Headaches, especially migraines

Increased sensitivity to pain

Inability to remember dreams

Alcohol and/or carbohydrate cravings   anxiety, panic attacks

Seasonal affective disorder (depression during winter)

How is serotonin made in the brain?

Serotonin is made in the brain from the amino acid tryptophan. An enzyme called hydroxylase in conjunction with vitamin B 6 and magnesium, converts tryptophan into 5-hydroxytryptophan (5HTP) which is then converted into Serotonin.

The other name for serotonin is 5-hydroxytryptamine.

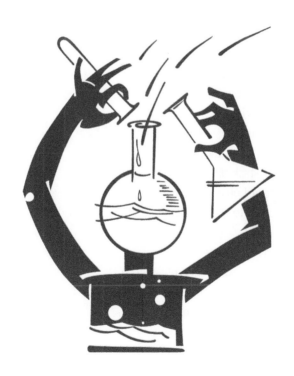

Dopamine – the chemical of focus, incentive, reward and pleasure

Dopamine is a powerful neurotransmitter found in areas of the brain concerned with pleasure and reward.

In the huge frontal lobes of the brain dopamine controls the flow of information from other areas of the brain. Dopamine disorders in this region of the brain can cause a decline in neurocognitive functions, especially attention, memory and problem-solving skills. Reduced dopamine concentrations in the frontal areas of the brain are thought to contribute to attention deficit disorder.

The symptoms that may be related to a deficiency in dopamine include:

- Depression
- Mental fatigue
- Loss of motivation
- Light-headedness
- Poor memory
- Poor concentration
- Routine-task difficulty
- Decreased physical activity
- Addiction to food, alcohol or other substances
- Cravings
- Excessive appetite
- Inability to experience pleasure
- Inability to be satisfied
- Inability to feel rewarded
- Tremors
- Low libido

Deficiency of dopamine

Deficiency of dopamine can lead to conditions including obesity, food and other addictions and sexual disorders. A severe deficiency of dopamine in specific areas of the brain causes Parkinson's disease.

The amino acids tyrosine and phenylalanine are the raw materials for the brain's production of dopamine. Phenylalanine is an amino acid that can be converted in the body to tyrosine, which in turn is used to synthesise the neurotransmitter dopamine.

Because tyrosine is converted into dopamine in the brain, it is often helpful for reducing symptoms of dopamine deficiency. Thus tyrosine can be helpful in addictive states, mental fatigue and depression. For similar reasons tyrosine helps to suppress the appetite and reduce food addiction.

Some antidepressant drugs increase the amount of dopamine in the brain.

dopamine

noradrenalin

Noradrenalin –
the chemical of drive, excitement and energy

This brain neurotransmitter is made from the amino acid tyrosine. Noradrenalin is a natural and powerful stimulant and excessive amounts can produce feelings of immense energy, invincibility, drive and euphoria. If a person takes cocaine or amphetamines this causes the body to be flooded with adrenalin and noradrenalin and this is why cocaine and speed are so addictive.

Adrenalin is a chemical that prepares the body for fight or flight if a person is faced with danger or a huge physical or mental challenge; in this situation adrenalin is adaptive and useful.

Conversely if the body releases large amounts of adrenalin when a person is not faced with a real danger or challenge, then it will cause a state of inappropriate and excessive stimulation. This can result in excess anxiety, stress, racing heartbeat, high blood pressure, chest pain, diarrhoea, sweating, muscle tension, agitation, shortness of breath and panic. The perceived threat is due to a chemical imbalance in the brain and body and is not real. This is very frightening and produces a feeling of being out of control. If severe, a panic attack may occur.

Abnormally low levels of noradrenalin in the brain produce extreme fatigue, apathetic depression and loss of drive and loss of interest. Some antidepressant drugs such as the SNRIs (Serotonin and Noradrenalin Reuptake Inhibitors) and the MAOIs (Mono Amine Oxidase Inhibitors) are able to increase the amount of adrenalin and noradrenalin in the brain.

Chapter Four

Antidepressant drugs

Modern day antidepressant drugs

The expression I like to use to describe the way antidepressant drugs work is – "they recharge the flat battery". Remember our analogy of the brain to a battery? – if your brain is flat or discharged, then antidepressant drugs will recharge your brain. Put another way, antidepressant drugs correct the chemical imbalance which causes your brain to go flat in the first place.

The chemicals that give the brain its energy are collectively called neurotransmitters and they are also called biogenic amines. The biogenic amines consist of dopamine, noradrenalin, adrenalin and serotonin.

All antidepressant drugs work by making these biogenic amines more available to relevant parts of the brain. So one could hypothesize that a deficiency of biogenic amines in the brain causes its energy to decrease and the "brain goes flat" – this supports the idea that depression and anxiety are caused by a deficiency or imbalance of biogenic amines in the brain. This deficiency of biogenic amines in the brain is the chemical imbalance I refer to that causes depression and anxiety.

Some people have a mental block about using drugs or anything chemical or unnatural to treat an illness. However if holistic medicine is required, this mental attitude can work against that person getting well. A more palatable or acceptable way for these people to view antidepressant drugs is to understand that they increase the availability and efficacy of naturally occurring body substances – namely the biogenic amines.

The use of antidepressant drugs has often been controversial in that they are commonly thought of as dangerous, addictive or a sign of weakness.

I have an old tattered book titled *"Lecture Notes on Psychiatry"* that I used during my years as a medical student. This book authored by Dr James Willis, was published in 1964, when the choices of antidepressant drugs were limited to two varieties. The author of this book, a well respected psychiatrist in London, gave me the impression that he thought that antidepressant drugs, although already widely prescribed, had not been proven to be effective and that clinical trials had shown conflicting results. He stated that depressive illness has a high rate of spontaneous remission (curing itself) and that the enthusiasm amongst doctors for prescribing antidepressant drugs was due to this factor.

In contrast the book titled *"Listening to Prozac"*, written by psychiatrist Dr Peter Kramer, and published in 1993, gives a very different outlook on antidepressant drugs. Prozac was the first of the class of antidepressant drugs known as Selective Serotonin Re-uptake Inhibitors (SSRIs), to be released into medical practice and this occurred in 1988. This book is a fascinating account of the hugely beneficial improvements that occurred in Dr Kramer's patients once they were commenced on Prozac. Dr Kramer explores the ethical and human issues that must be explored to make the decision to start a patient on an antidepressant drug. Overall Dr Kramer is a protagonist of this new breed of antidepressant drugs that have been made famous by Prozac. His book is a literary masterpiece and made it to the top of the New York Times best seller list and I highly recommend this book as reading material for those fascinated by the topics of emotional illness, the pursuit of happiness and psychology.

Frequently Ask Questions

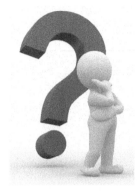

Question – *Are antidepressant drugs addictive?*

Answer

No they are not addictive; however if you have been taking them for several years it may take up to 6 months to gradually come off them. The important thing is to lower the dose of the drug very gradually; for example you start by taking the drug every second day or on alternate days you take the full dose and then a half dose. There are many ways to reduce the dose gradually and you need to work with your doctor to formulate a plan for this. Always see your doctor regularly while reducing the dose

Question – *Once I have been on antidepressant drugs, should I aim to eventually come off these drugs altogether?*

Answer

This depends on the cause of your emotional illness and the answer will vary between individual patients. If your depression has been caused by the loss of something important in your life, once you have come to terms with this loss, and feel emotionally stable and happy, you can try to come off the drugs gradually. Similarly if your depression has been caused by stress due to external or relationship problems, once these issues are resolved, you will be able to gradually wean yourself off the antidepressant drug.

If you have inherited the genes for depression and/ or anxiety it will be harder to stay off antidepressant drugs forever. This is because in this situation the drug is treating the cause of your depressive illness which is a chemical imbalance caused by the type of genes you have inherited. Thus inherited depression is not caused by life events such as loss or stress which are often temporary events. Conversely the genetic form of depression and anxiety is often permanent because the chemical imbalance, being genetic in origin, is permanent. Many people with genetic depression feel so much better and more normal on antidepressant drugs and when they try to stop them, their chemical imbalance recurs bringing back the emotional illness. In this situation it may be better to accept your illness, in the same way that people accept the fact that they need drugs to control inherited asthma, heart disease or epilepsy etc. The understanding that genetic depression is a chemical imbalance and thus beyond the help of psychology and counselling alone, removes the misconceived stigma that antidepressants are bad or a sign of weakness. It is quite safe and logical to stay on antidepressant drugs long term in the case of chronic genetic depressive illness.

Question – If I wish to come off my antidepressant medication what is the best way to do this?

Answer

First of all tell your doctor who will explain the best way to do this, as antidepressant drugs should not be stopped abruptly. If you suddenly stop them you will probably experience unpleasant symptoms such as headache, dizziness, depression, anxiety, nausea and pins and needles. It is best to come off antidepressants very gradually by tapering off the dose. This can take up to 6 months and various schedules can be used such as taking your medication every second day for a month and then taking your medication every third day. But do not do this without your own doctor's supervision. Make sure you avoid alcohol whilst coming off your antidepressants and maintain a healthy diet and lifestyle and keep taking your natural supplements.

Question – *Are antidepressant drugs dangerous?*

Answer

Generally speaking antidepressant drugs are very safe but like all drugs they must be prescribed carefully and with precautions. If one compares the side effects of drugs that are commonly prescribed for long term use such as anti-inflammatory drugs, steroids, some antibiotics, some diuretics, immunosuppressant drugs and some cholesterol lowering drugs, the side effects of antidepressant drugs are far less dangerous. Doctors are well aware of the precautions of prescribing antidepressant drugs and this is particularly so in patients who are agitated and/or at risk of suicide. In these cases some types of antidepressant drugs can increase agitation or the risk of suicide and in such cases the patient must be supervised at all times until they are emotionally stable. In overdose situations the more modern types of antidepressant drugs are less dangerous than the older types such as the tricyclic drugs and the monoamine oxidase inhibitors.

Question – *Do antidepressant drugs have a lot of side effects?*

Answer

Most possible side effects occur during the first 2 weeks of treatment and will disappear after the drug becomes effective.

If antidepressant drugs are incorrectly prescribed, potential side effects will be worse. It is important to tailor the initial dose of the antidepressant drug to suit the severity of the depression and/or anxiety. In most cases the initial or starting dose of the antidepressant drug should be the lowest possible and over a period of 2 weeks the dose should be increased to the required or maintenance dose. By starting with the smallest dose, side effects can often be avoided. Ask your doctor to consider this fact.

Question – *Will I still be "me" whilst taking antidepressant drugs?*

Answer

Yes you will still be yourself whilst taking antidepressant drugs and indeed if you have lost your old happy go lucky self, you should find that you will gradually return to that happier self after several weeks to months. Antidepressant drugs if given to a person who really needs them may allow a person to grow and develop in a more positive way as they remove the emotional problems that have held them back for years. This is particularly so in people who have inherited genetic chronic depression and/or anxiety, because the correction of the chemical imbalance in their brain may improve their personality in a way that they enjoy life much more. For example they may become more relaxed, more expressive, more energetic, more confident, more courageous, more assertive and more extroverted. Thus we could say that in such people the antidepressant drug has enabled them to become more like the personality they had wanted to be but found difficult to achieve.

Question – *Is taking antidepressant drugs a sign of weakness and should I resist taking them?*

Answer

The answer is no, the need to take an antidepressant drug is not a sign of weakness or giving in. Indeed the truth is that it may make you stronger and more functional and thus you will be able to achieve more in your life. If you achieve more in your own life this will not only help you but will help others too. Taking an antidepressant drug may be essential either to cope with the stress of a temporary and intolerable situation or a chronic chemical imbalance in your brain. Remember you cannot overcome a severe chemical imbalance in your brain with positive thoughts and will power alone; it's like a "catch 22 situation"; the chemical imbalance causes the negative thoughts and emotions and these negative thoughts will aggravate your chemical imbalance.

Question – *Will antidepressant drugs slow me down?*

Answer

Most types of antidepressant drugs do not slow you down mentally or physically, especially if large doses are avoided, and it is usually possible to avoid the need for large doses on a long term basis. Many people find that once the antidepressant drug relieves their fatigue, muscle pain and anxiety, they are able to become more motivated and become a lot more efficient. The symptoms of depression and anxiety if untreated will slow you down, as they are very distracting and use up a lot of wasted energy.

Question – *Do antidepressant drugs work the same way as sedative drugs?*

Answer

No they are very different in their mechanism of action to sedative drugs. Sedative drugs, such as those belonging to the benzodiazepine family of drugs, do not correct the chemical imbalance in the brain that causes depression and/or anxiety. Sedative drugs work by suppressing and controlling the symptoms of anxiety. Examples of the benzodiazepine family of drugs are diazepam (also known under the brand name of Valium), lorazepam, oxazepam (also known under the brand name of Serepax), clobazam, bromazepam, alprazolam (also known under the brand of Xanax) and Temazepam. These types of sedative drugs can be addictive or habit forming and ideally their use should be minimised and temporary.

Xanax is effective for panic anxiety. Xanax does not cause sedation like some of the other benzodiazepine sedatives do, and has fewer side effects. Xanax is, however, addictive and short acting and thus it is difficult to get off it.

Buspirone is another type of sedative drug.

Sedative drugs may be used by people prone to panic attacks but remember they are relieving the symptoms only and will not prevent more anxiety and/or panic attacks. Antidepressant drugs are far less habit forming and in most cases can prevent anxiety and panic attacks. Sedative drugs and sleeping tablets are often prescribed to patients who suffer with insomnia or anxiety/panic attacks, and in many of these patients an antidepressant drug would be more effective and less addictive.

Question – *Can antidepressant drugs be taken with hormone therapy?*

Answer

Yes they can and if the depression is caused partly by hormonal imbalances it is much more effective to try hormone therapy either alone or with antidepressant drugs. The hormone therapy and the antidepressant can have a synergistic effect – in other words they help each other to more quickly and effectively stop the depression and/or anxiety.

Question – *Can antidepressant drugs be used at the same time as natural therapies?*

Answer

Ideally all patients with a depressive or anxiety illness should be given a program that incorporates specific natural therapies and a brain boosting diet.

Generally speaking the use of natural therapies along with a brain boosting diet will allow smaller doses of antidepressant drugs to be much more effective. Natural therapies will often prevent the need to use large doses of antidepressant drugs on a long term basis.

There are a few contra-indications to combining certain nutritional supplements or herbs with antidepressant drugs and these are –

The herb hypericum (also known as St John's Wort) cannot be given with any antidepressant drugs.

The amino acid tyrosine cannot be given with stimulant types of antidepressant drugs such as monoamine oxidase inhibitors (MAOIs).

Always check with your own doctor or naturopath first to avoid interactions or phone the Health Advisory Service on (02) 4655 8855.

What are the choices of antidepressant drugs?

Tricyclic antidepressants

Tricyclic antidepressants were first discovered in the 1950s and have been used extensively worldwide to alleviate disorders such as depression, anxiety, obsessive compulsive disorder and panic attacks. They are also used to help those with insomnia and can reduce the pain of post herpetic neuralgia. Some people find that they are useful for reducing migraine and tension headaches and fibromyalgia.

Examples of tricyclic antidepressant drugs are imipramine, amitriptyline, desipramine, nortriptyline, doxepin, mianserin, clomipramine, lofepramine and trazodone.

Advantages of Tricyclic antidepressants

The tricyclic drugs are highly effective antidepressants and 60 to 70% of patients will respond well after several weeks of treatment.

They are particularly good for:

Poor sleep

Anxiety

Panic attacks

Bladder irritability and overactivity

Nocturnal urinary frequency

Nervous diarrhoea

Reduced appetite

Disadvantages of Tricyclic antidepressants

Tricyclic antidepressant drugs not only affect the brain but also affect the nervous control of many automatic bodily functions.

This can cause side effects such as:

Palpitations and a racing heartbeat

Dry mouth

Blurred vision

Constipation

Urinary retention

Mild tremor

Increased sweating

Postural hypotension (the blood pressure drops if you stand up too rapidly)

They can also cause weight gain and mild sedation in some people; but if small doses are used to start with these side effects can be minimised.

If a depressed patient attempts to overdose with tricyclic drugs, this can result in toxic and dangerous effects on the heart.

Monoamine Oxidase Inhibitors (MAOIs)

The Monoamine Oxidase Inhibitor (MAOI) drugs are very effective and powerful antidepressants and act by increasing the brain's levels of the stimulating neurotransmitters noradrenalin and dopamine.

Examples of MAOI drugs are Nardil (phenelzine) and Parnate (tranylcypromine).

Advantages of MAOIs

Work quickly – within 24 to 48 hours of initiating therapy

Exert a stimulating effect on the brain

Increase mental and physical energy

May work where all other antidepressant drugs have failed

Can be excellent for people who suffer with depression associated with obsessional or hypochondriacal features

Disadvantages of MAOIs

Side effects may occur in some people such as

Insomnia

Appetite changes

A special low amine diet must be followed otherwise serious side effects can occur if foods containing tyramine or dopamine are eaten. These serious side effects can include high blood pressure, stroke and severe headache.

Other drugs must not be mixed with MAOIs unless first checking with your doctor and pharmacist, as dangerous drug interactions can occur with pethidine, amphetamines, ephedrine, pseudoephedrine, levodopa and several others.

If the low amine diet is followed carefully, then the MAOI drugs are quite safe.

The low amine diet excludes foods high in amines such as Chianti wine, ripe figs, broad beans, flava beans, fermented foods, pickled herrings, yeast extract, partially decomposed foods such as game or aged meat, mature cheeses and several others. When you receive your MAOI tablets you receive a list of all the foods you must avoid whilst taking these tablets. The list is not huge and most patients do not find it hard to stick to the required low amine diet

Selective Serotonin Reuptake Inhibitors (SSRIs)

These drugs increase the amount of the neurotransmitter serotonin in the brain.

The first Selective Serotonin Reuptake Inhibitor (SSRI) drug was called Prozac and was released in December 1987. The introduction of the SSRI drugs revolutionised the practice of psychiatry, as for the first time in history doctors had a class of antidepressant drugs that were very effective, relatively free of side effects, relatively safe and specific in action.

Dr Kramer, the author of the best selling book *"Listening to Prozac"*, describes Prozac as a "designed drug which is sleek and high tech". Dr Kramer describes the SSRI class of antidepressant drugs as "clean drugs", meaning they tend to have fewer side effects than the Tricyclic or Monoamine Oxidase Inhibitor (MAOI) class of antidepressant drugs.

Examples of SSRIs drugs are Citalopram, Escitalopram, Fluoxetine (Prozac), Paroxetine, Fluvoxamine and Sertraline.

Since the introduction of the SSRI drugs there have been more improvements in the design of antidepressants and we now have drugs which not only increase serotonin levels in the brain, but also increase levels of other neurotransmitters such as noradrenalin. These newer drugs are known as Serotonin and Noradrenalin Reuptake Inhibitors (SNRIs). The SNRI drugs have become very trusted and widely prescribed by the medical profession.

Some doctors find that the SNRIs are more effective, especially for people with chronic genetic depression.

SNRI drugs are effective for people who suffer with social anxiety disorder where they feel uncomfortable in social situations or crowds. An example of an SNRI drug is called venlafaxine (EfexorXR).

Another type of antidepressant drug increases the release of serotonin and noradrenalin in the brain, the best known one being called mirtazapine (Avanza).

A newer type of antidepressant drug which increases only noradrenalin in the brain is called reboxetine. It is highly effective in severe depression but there are some precautions in its use in those with glaucoma, high blood pressure, heart disease, epilepsy or a tendency to manic episodes.

Another SNRI antidepressant drug called Duloxetine has been released onto the Australian market with treatment indications for not only depression and anxiety but also stress urinary incontinence, painful neuropathy and the pain of fibromyalgia. This is not surprising because chronic stress can manifest in the body as psychosomatic disorders such as fibromyalgia, headaches and backache. In such cases the patient may be unaware that anxiety is causing their physical pain. The fact that an antidepressant drug can relieve physical pain, illustrates just how powerfully chronic stress upsets the control of muscular contractions and blood flow to the muscles throughout the body.

Advantages of SSRIs and SNRIs

Highly effective in relieving the symptoms of depression and/or anxiety

Can reduce/prevent being excessively sensitive to loss or rejection

Can prevent anxiety and panic attacks

Can be effective for eating disorders such as anorexia or bulimia

Can reduce attention deficit disorder

Can reduce obsessive compulsive disorders

Can make you more adventurous

Can increase the ability to experience pleasure

Can make you more extroverted and social

Can make you less inhibited

Can make you feel more secure inside yourself

Can make you more assertive and confident

Generally speaking, the SSRI class of drugs has fewer side effects than other classes of antidepressant drugs

There is no need to follow a special diet whilst taking this class of drugs and small amounts of alcohol can be consumed socially whist taking these drugs.

Overdoses of the SSRI drugs are far less dangerous than overdoses of the Tricyclic or MAOI drugs.

Disadvantages of SSRI and SNRI Drugs

All drugs can have side effects and with antidepressant drugs these side effects usually occur in the first 2 to 4 weeks after commencing them. If the smallest possible doses are used initially, the side effects are usually minimal. I have found that if a patient really needs antidepressant drugs, they usually do not get significant side effects if small doses are used to start with.

Possible side effects include

Fatigue

Headaches, but in some cases headaches will reduce as the tension is relieved

Reduced sex drive and inability to orgasm

Nightmares

Increased sweating

Digestive disturbances such as nausea or abdominal cramps – this can be reduced by taking the medication with food. Antacids may help to reduce side effects.

Skin rashes

Elevation of blood pressure

Increased heart rate

Bleeding disorders – bruising, nose bleeds, vaginal bleeding, gastro-intestinal bleeding

Low blood sodium

Restlessness of the limbs whilst sitting or standing still

Agitation in those with bipolar illness (manic depression)

If prescribed inappropriately, may increase the risk of suicide

Liver inflammation

Weight loss or weight gain

Increased risk of osteoporosis

Talk to your doctor

Because depression, anxiety and inability to cope with stress are such common problems, the study of substances which favourably influence the brain's biochemistry will increase enormously. Although true happiness cannot be found in a drug or supplement it is nevertheless true that these things can help human beings to cope with the difficulties of life. They can raise the threshold at which stress affects us adversely, numb the pain of rejection and failure, and enable us to be more detached and objective about our problems.

If you think that you may be depressed, talk to your local doctor. Your own GP may be very good at counselling or can set up a mental health care plan for you.

Your own GP will know if you need antidepressant drugs and/or need to see a specialist psychiatrist. Psychiatrists are fully qualified medical doctors, who have completed post-graduate study in the field of mental and emotional problems. A referral is needed from your GP to see a psychiatrist. A Medicare rebate is available for visits to a psychiatrist, and some may even bulk bill in cases of financial difficulty.

Case history

P auline had been one of my patients for years and had always been very sensitive and easily upset by criticism or rejection from others. After menopause she became depressed, could not sleep and was unable to keep her job. We tried a tricyclic antidepressant and she did not really respond, finding that after 4 months she still felt very down and fatigued. We decided to stop the tricyclic antidepressant for 4 weeks and then start her on the selective serotonin reuptake inhibitor drug called Aropax. After 3 months on Aropax Pauline decided that she still felt depressed although she was now sleeping normally. She said that she felt like she was in a "chemical straightjacket" and wanted to come off the Aropax. So we opted for a more natural approach of fish oil and magnesium and she went to counselling sessions and support groups to learn how to become more assertive.

Pauline slowly improved, but did not entirely recover. Pauline still found that she was prone to depression and anxiety and was not able to return to work. She found that she was still overly sensitive to criticism from her son and her ex husband who tried to make her feel guilty.

I said to Pauline, "Why don't we try a new type of antidepressant drug to see if we can really get your brain chemistry balanced?" I thought that Pauline was suffering from the type of depression due to a lack of the neurotransmitters noradrenalin and dopamine, and not a lack of serotonin. This was because the other drugs I had tried, namely the SSRI and the tricyclic drug increase serotonin levels, but in her case this had not worked.

Pauline was keen to try this as she knew she had a chemical imbalance and she had tried everything she could to overcome it and yet it persisted. She said to me "I take after my mother who was depressed most of her life and I look like her and I react like her even though I try not to; it must be in my genes". I said yes you are right; a chemical imbalance is often inherited and needs to be fixed with another chemical. Pauline said "My poor mother was dominated by a controlling and overly critical husband and I don't want to be like my mother; she got more depressed and helpless as she aged". I replied "Well Pauline it is such a relief that you live in a time where modern pharmacology has a solution for you because in the past many people with these imbalances never found relief".

I started Pauline on the MAOI drug called Parnate which increases the brain levels of the neurotransmitters dopamine and noradrenalin. After one week Pauline felt completely different – she had more energy and was motivated and cheerful. After 3 months on the Parnate, Pauline was really enjoying life more than she had been able to in years and she was no longer overly sensitive to the more powerful members of her family. She was now able to cope with their criticisms and moodiness with detachment and confidence. Pauline returned to her old work place and her work mates were surprised by her new found wellbeing and confidence. She had decided not to tell anyone she was taking antidepressants, which in many cases is a wise move, as many people do not understand these medications.

The case history of Pauline demonstrates that it can take time and some trial and error with antidepressant drugs to find the correct drug to overcome the specific chemical imbalance that may be causing an emotional illness in an individual. Just because one antidepressant drug fails, one should not give up on finding a solution to overcoming depression with other drugs or strategies.

Chapter Five

Natural treatments for depression

Nutritional deficiencies and imbalances can cause deficiencies of neurotransmitters such as noradrenalin, dopamine and serotonin. Nutritional deficiencies can also result in adverse physical changes in the brain, which can lead to mood and cognition problems. The pioneers of the nutritional treatment of mental and emotional disorders were Dr Abram Hoffer (Canada) and Carl Pfeiffer (USA) and during the 20th century they developed nutritional protocols for many nervous problems.

Hypericum

The herb hypericum, also known as Saint John's wort, has been used since ancient Greek times as a remedy for nervous complaints. The clinical success of hypericum extracts for the treatment of patients with depression has been confirmed in a large number of placebo-controlled double-blind studies. One great benefit of hypericum is that in the doses used in humans it is usually free of side effects. Allergic reactions can occur in those who are generally allergic to herbs and may manifest as photo-sensitivity rashes when exposed to sunshine.

Hypericum is thought to exert its antidepressant and mood elevating effect in a similar way to the Mono-Amine-Oxidase Inhibitor (MAOI) antidepressant drugs. In other words it is able to inhibit the enzymes that break down the brain chemicals noradrenalin and serotonin.

Most studies demonstrating that hypericum is an effective antidepressant have used a standardised extract of the herb which gives a dose of 900mcg total hypericin three times daily. This is equivalent to tablets containing 300mg of a 6:1 extract of the herb. One 300mg tablet, three times daily, has been found to be the generally effective therapeutic dose, although some people will find that they only need to take one or two tablets daily.

High levels of scientific and clinical evidence have shown that hypericum is a first line treatment in the management of mild to moderate depression.

Another interesting benefit of hypericum is that several studies have demonstrated its pronounced inhibition of multiplication of some types of viruses, particularly retroviruses, such as the human immunodeficiency virus which causes AIDS. Hypericum is combined with all the B group vitamins and minerals in one tablet called StressEze for added effect.

Warning – Hypericum should not be taken with certain drugs because adverse interactions may occur – these include other antidepressant drugs, blood thinners and the oral contraceptive pill. Check with your own doctor before taking hypericum containing products.

Mineral supplements

Mineral deficiencies are common in many parts of the world, even in so called well fed societies, and are more common in depressed people who often have a poor diet.

Mineral deficiencies can lead to impaired production of the brain's neurotransmitters.

The mineral magnesium, along with vitamin B 6, is required for the conversion of the amino acid tryptophan, into the happy chemical serotonin.

Depression associated with irritability and agitation, may be part of a magnesium deficiency syndrome. Magnesium is often called the **"great relaxer"** as it helps to reduce nervous and muscular tension and promotes deep restful sleep. Magnesium when taken regularly can also help to prevent and reduce the symptoms of a panic attack.

Zinc is another mineral that is commonly deficient in modern processed food. Zinc deficiency can lead to appetite disturbances, fatigue and reduced libido, all of which can be symptoms of depression.

Selenium is frequently deficient in Australian soils and thus in foods grown in these soils. A 5-week double blind cross over study, involving 50 volunteers who received a daily supplement containing either selenium or placebo found that selenium was associated with improvement in mood. The lower their initial dietary selenium intake, the more the mood improved. Selenium is also important for immune function, and severe depression can lead to an impaired immune system.

The minerals manganese and zinc can also help to reduce the symptoms of dizziness and light headedness that can be part of depression and anxiety.

Unstable blood sugar levels can produce mental fogginess, dizziness and unpleasant moods such as anxiety and irritability. They can also lead to fatigue, sugar cravings and disturbances of appetite. Those suffering with anxiety-depression syndromes often have poor diets and consume large amounts of refined sugar and caffeine, which destabilise blood sugar levels. This can worsen their symptoms of nervous dysfunction. Eating sugar gives temporary relief from depression or anxiety, but these symptoms worsen as the blood sugar level falls again later. Supplements of the minerals chromium and magnesium can greatly reduce this problem and reduce cravings for sweets or other high carbohydrate foods.

B group vitamins

Many people who live and work in high stress situations that demand a high level of performance or patience will find that supplemental doses of the B group vitamins help them to cope. I have found that best results are obtained by combining **all** the B group vitamins with their synergistic co-factors, which are choline, inositol, folic acid and biotin. This combination is found in most B vitamin tablets and also in the StressEze tablets.

The brain has a high requirement for B vitamins (especially B6) and is unable to manufacture adequate amounts of the neurotransmitters serotonin and dopamine without them. These neurotransmitters control mental energy, concentration, memory and sleep patterns. Deficiencies of the B group vitamins can lead to depressive symptoms and dysfunction of the spinal cord and nerves.

Magnesium

I have used magnesium supplements extensively over more than 30 years of medical practice and have found that it is a great balancer for the nervous system. Magnesium is a mineral that is required in greater amounts in those with stress and anxiety. This is because magnesium exerts a calming effect upon the central nervous system and helps nerves and muscles to relax. When we are stressed our bodies use up far greater quantities of magnesium, and magnesium deficient people overreact to minor stress.

Magnesium can often greatly reduce or completely alleviate many of the symptoms of stress and anxiety and will help those with the following problems:

> Muscle cramps and muscle pain
> Fibromyalgia
> Whole body tremor

Muscle twitches

Poor sleep

High blood pressure

Racing heartbeat and palpitations

Abdominal cramps and irritable bowel

Urinary frequency

Asthma attacks

Migraine and tension headaches

Panic attacks

I use a tablet which combines 4 different types of magnesium salts – namely magnesium phosphate, magnesium aspartate, magnesium orotate and magnesium amino acid chelate. The dose is 2 tablets twice daily and this provides 292 mg of pure elemental magnesium. I avoid magnesium supplements containing magnesium oxide, as this form of magnesium salt is not well absorbed from the gut into the blood stream or cells.

You can also get an Ultra potent magnesium powder which contains 4 different types of magnesium and the amino acid taurine. This powder is stirred into water or juice and best taken one hour before retiring. Taurine is also a calming agent and relaxes the nerves and the muscles thereby improving the effect of magnesium. Supplements of magnesium and taurine can help those with migraine headaches, tension headaches, fibromyalgia, muscle tension and difficult to control epilepsy. Magnesium supplements can safely be taken along with anticonvulsant drugs or antidepressant drugs.

Magnesium supplements are excellent for those under stress caused by a high physical or mental workload.

For more information on Magnesium, see the book titled *Magnesium The Miracle Mineral – You won't believe the difference it makes to your health!*

Case histories

One day a 49 year old high powered male executive who ran his own business came to my office. I noticed that he was flushed in the face which proved to be due to high and poorly controlled blood pressure. His arms, legs and face had a fine tremor and his reflexes were very brisk. He complained of poor sleep and an inability to relax and unwind and he said that he was on "overdrive" all the time. He had suffered with a nervous collapse in the past due to excess work load and trying to please all his customers. He was a very nice person who was a perfectionist and tried to attend to every detail to keep his customers happy.

I suggested that we give him four magnesium tablets a day and he was happy to try this safe and simple treatment as drugs had been only partially effective for him and he did not want to be slowed down by anything. He returned to see me after two weeks of this magnesium therapy and was amazed by the improvement in his wellbeing. He felt normal again and was relaxed and coping much better. His sleep was getting better and his tremor had disappeared. Even better his blood pressure had come down to normal. This gentleman continues to take his magnesium supplement and is now one of my greatest fans. He has nicknamed himself "mag man"

A 52 year old executive came to see me complaining of leg pain, very poor sleep and problems maintaining an erection. He felt stressed from his workload and lack of sleep, as most nights he only got one to two hours of sleep when he would be woken by muscle cramps and pain in his legs. He had been like this for 15 years and had not been able to find relief from any pain killers or other drugs. Physical examination and tests did not reveal any problems with the circulation of blood to his legs, brain or heart and he was not diabetic. His cholesterol levels and blood pressure were normal.

I asked myself "Could this be a magnesium deficiency?" Blood tests showed his magnesium levels to be at the lower limit of the normal range.

I prescribed an ultrapotent magnesium powder in a dose of one teaspoon in water before retiring. This provided a total elemental amount of 400mg magnesium per teaspoon.

This man did not respond as quickly as the previous case; however after 6 weeks he was sleeping much better and was delighted to be achieving 4 to 5 hours of unbroken sleep for the first time in 15 years! He no longer suffered any leg pain or muscle cramps and felt more relaxed. After 8 weeks he found that his erections were better and lasted longer and this is due to the fact that magnesium dilates the arteries which supply blood to the penis.

L – Tryptophan

This is an essential amino acid meaning it must be obtained from the diet or from supplements because the body cannot manufacture its own supply. See table on page 79 for food sources of tryptophan.

L – Tryptophan is converted into the neurotransmitter serotonin in the nervous system and if adequate amounts of tryptophan are not present in the diet, a deficiency of serotonin can occur. This can result in depression, anxiety and insomnia.

Advantages of tryptophan supplements

May exert a natural calming effect

May reduce aggressive behaviour

May reduce binge eating in eating disorders (such as bulimia)

May relieve insomnia

May relieve restless legs, especially if it is combined with supplements of magnesium and fish oil

Doses vary from one to two grams at night or one gram twice daily. Tryptophan supplements should not be taken at the same time as food containing protein, as this will reduce its absorption into the brain. Take the tryptophan with a protein free beverage such as milk free tea, fruit juice or fruit.

Smaller doses of tryptophan which are available over the counter will not help those with depression or anxiety symptoms. To get the effective dose of 2 grams daily, you will need a doctor's prescription. This is because even though tryptophan is a natural non-toxic substance, it was falsely maligned by a contaminated batch of tryptophan made in Japan in the late 1980s. Ever since this false scare, tryptophan has not been available over the counter in adequate strength.

Tyrosine

Tyrosine is an amino acid found in protein foods such as milk and cheese, chicken, fish, almonds, bananas and avocados. Tyrosine can also be made in the body from another amino acid called phenylalanine.

Tyrosine is required for several vitally important functions in the body and these include:

- **Production of brain chemicals**. Tyrosine is the raw material needed for the manufacture of the important brain neurotransmitters called dopamine and noradrenalin; these neurotransmitters regulate mood and emotions.

Low dopamine and noradrenalin levels have been linked with

Food cravings (particularly for carbohydrate)

Excessive appetite

Reduced ability to achieve satisfaction

Reduced ability to experience pleasure

Reduced concentration and mental drive

- **Thyroid hormone production**. Tyrosine is used by the thyroid gland to manufacture the thyroid hormones T4 and T3. T4 consists of tyrosine bound to four iodine molecules and T3 consists of tyrosine bound to three iodine molecules. Thyroid hormones regulate the body's metabolic rate and energy production; thus getting adequate tyrosine is essential to control your weight. Tyrosine is part of the Metabocel formula for weight loss. Tyrosine can be an excellent antidepressant for those with sluggish metabolism, excess food cravings and weight excess.

- **Melanin production**. Tyrosine is required for the production of the pigment melanin. Melanin gives hair and skin attractive colours.

- **Natural pain relieving substances**. Tyrosine is needed for the body's production of enkephalins, which are substances that have natural pain relieving effects in the body.

Why would it be beneficial to supplement with tyrosine?

A study carried out by Dr Alan Gelenberg of the Harvard Medical School showed clearly that a lack of the amino acid tyrosine resulted in a deficiency of the brain neurotransmitter noradrenalin. This deficiency occurred at certain locations in the brain, which relate specifically to mood disorders.

Tyrosine can be an excellent and safe natural antidepressant and in general exerts a stimulating effect. Tyrosine can lift the mood and improve concentration and mental drive.

Some people have a higher requirement for tyrosine than others. High workload, stress, poor diet, poor appetite and poor digestion, as well as genetic factors may be responsible for this. Poor protein digestion is common in people with irritable bowel syndrome, abdominal bloating and those taking antacid medication. Chronic stress often impairs digestion and absorption of protein because it disrupts the production of digestive enzymes and stomach acid. Neurotransmitters in the brain can become depleted due to stress, alcohol, caffeine and sugar. Each of these factors increases the requirement for tyrosine. Sometimes tyrosine is referred to as a "mood food" because it is a protein supplement that can improve mood.

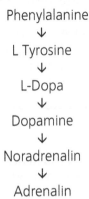

Phenylalanine
↓
L Tyrosine
↓
L-Dopa
↓
Dopamine
↓
Noradrenalin
↓
Adrenalin

Pathways of neurotransmitter production in the brain

Tyrosine supplementation may provide the following benefits

- Improved concentration and alertness
- Better memory
- More motivation
- Increased ability to experience satisfaction and pleasure
- Reduction in depression
- Reduction of appetite in those with eating disorders, particularly overeating
- More efficient metabolism, due to improved thyroid hormone production
- Improved energy levels

Some people battling with drug and/or alcohol addiction find that tyrosine helps them to detoxify and reduce their cravings. It has been used successfully to help people overcome a cocaine addiction.

How to take tyrosine

Tyrosine is best taken at least 30 minutes before meals, two or three times daily. The recommended dose is 1 to 2 grams, two or three times daily. Some people may need higher doses than this, so work with your health care practitioner to increase the dose, if lower doses are ineffective.

Tyrosine can be taken in the form of a pure white powder and is tasteless and odourless. This powder can be eaten off a spoon or stirred into water or juice.

For more information contact the
Health Advisory Service
on (02) 4655 8855.

Cautions when taking tyrosine supplements

Tyrosine supplements must not be used by people taking monoamine oxidase inhibitor (MAOI) antidepressant medications. Tyrosine can cause a severe rise in blood pressure in people taking these medications.

If you have high blood pressure or manic depression, check with your doctor before taking tyrosine.

If you have a malignant melanoma, don't take tyrosine unless you check with your doctor first.

Dopamine and obesity

New research shows that the pleasure of eating is due to the release in the brain of the neurotransmitter dopamine. Researchers found that in overweight persons the consumption of an equivalent amount of chocolate milk shake caused less dopamine to be released than in subjects who were not overweight.

In some overweight persons there is a gene that causes less dopamine to be released. The overweight persons could have a genetically based deficiency in the pleasure they get from eating and this makes them eat more to achieve satisfaction. More food is required to get the same amount of dopamine released, and thus the same amount of pleasure, compared to non overweight persons. Adequate pleasure from eating is called satiety.

Previously it was thought that obesity was only due to behaviour – in other words eating too much food and not enough exercise. Although this is partly true, we now know that this concept is far too simplistic. Our relationship with food is influenced by our genes and the chemicals that our genes control, especially dopamine release in the brain. Thus supplements such as tyrosine, which increase the production of the brain's dopamine, can reduce appetite and increase the amount of pleasure gained from a certain amount of food.

SAMe

SAMe (pronounced "Sammy") is the abbreviation for S-adenosyl-L-methionine. SAMe is a natural chemical manufactured by the liver and is required throughout the body for a chemical process called methylation. Methylation is one of the last chemical reactions in the production of the brain neurotransmitters serotonin, dopamine and noradrenalin.

There are no foods that have high SAMe levels and our liver must make it from the amino acid methionine, which is found in many protein foods. Good sources of methionine are – eggs, dairy products, liver and seafood.

You need a healthy liver because creating SAMe requires multiple steps in the liver cells and other co-factor nutrients, such as vitamin B12, vitamin B6 and folate to complete. Folate is found in fresh vegetables and vitamin B 12 is found in animal sources of protein such as meat, seafood, dairy products and eggs. By improving your liver function and your diet, you should be able to increase the production of SAMe. This would theoretically improve the metabolism of serotonin, dopamine and noradrenalin in your brain, exerting a natural antidepressant effect. Some studies suggest that SAMe may slow down the breakdown of these neurotransmitters, allowing them to work longer.

Some research has indicated that non-depressed and depressed people who take SAMe supplements have higher overall levels of serotonin, dopamine and noradrenalin but this is difficult to confirm. In research on treating depression, the positive effects of SAMe have sometimes been impressive. These studies, however, have been small, so it is difficult to determine which type of depression will benefit most from this supplement. High dose SAMe supplements are relatively expensive and often equally good results are obtained just by improving your liver function.

The liver and your state of mind

You may have heard of the term "lily-livered".

You may remember it from Shakespeare's play *Macbeth* or when someone used the term to describe a person who becomes frightened easily.

The ancient Greeks would sacrifice an animal before they went into battle with the enemy, and if the animal's liver was red it was a good sign; however, if the animal's liver was pale it was considered a bad omen.

The term Lily-livered is colloquially used to describe someone who

Has no courage

Cannot fight back when attacked

Spooks easily

Has "no balls"

Metaphorically speaking the liver is the site of anger – in other words it stores anger – thus the term "liverish" is often used to describe a grumpy, disgruntled person. I must admit that there is some truth in this because many of my patients feel more cheerful and positive when they improve their liver function.

If a person becomes very frightened or fearful, the body releases large amounts of the hormone adrenalin to prepare the body physiologically for a good fight. Adrenalin causes the blood vessels to constrict, which causes blood to be pushed out of the liver into the systemic circulation so that more blood is available to the heart and muscles. This is obviously needed if you have a good fight on your hands! When blood is taken from the liver during this adrenalin reaction, the liver becomes pale – thus the term "lily-livered" can be used physiologically to describe a frightened person.

It is interesting to think about the emotional state of those with a fatty liver, as in this common condition the liver becomes pale because it is infiltrated with fat. The fat reduces the blood spaces in the liver and because fat is a pale white to yellowish colour this gives the appearance of a "lily liver".

Courage and mood is not only influenced by your state of mind; your resistance to stress and what you feel you can cope with, has a lot to do with your physical health.

This curious phrase "lily-livered", gives us food for thought and the possibility that the foods we eat may influence our ability to cope with stress.

So by eating plenty of liver cleansing foods – such as fresh raw fruits and vegetables, fresh green leafy herbs, fresh raw juices and seeds and nuts, will help us to feel physically and mentally prepared for stress and challenging situations.

Environmental chemicals can make your brain toxic

The human brain is a fatty organ and fat-soluble toxic chemicals can get into the brain and accumulate for this reason. This is particularly so if exposure to such chemicals involves a large dose or chronic repeated exposure.

Many fat-soluble chemicals are made from petrochemicals (petroleum based) and are found in commonly used everyday products. These chemicals adversely affect the function of the brain and can result in mental fuzziness, mental fatigue, headaches and mood disorders.

Work places, homes and offices can have air with unhealthy levels of toxic brain chemicals.

These include such things as

> Air fresheners and aerosols
> Deodorisers
> Pesticides
> Insecticides
> Anti-fungal and anti-mould cleansers
> Carpet cleaners
> Solvents
> Thinners
> Varnish
> Paints
> Detergents

New homes have fixtures, carpets, paints and fittings that outgas for several years and can be toxic if people spend most of their time indoors.

These strong smelling chemicals emit fumes known as volatile organic compounds (VOCs). Once inhaled, VOCs find their way into your vulnerable brain.

Indoor plants have been found to be effective at removing VOCs from the air. For one averaged sized home, six indoor plants have been shown to be effective.

Try to avoid such toxic chemicals or minimise their use. Where possible use organic, non-toxic and bio-degradable cleaning agents. Keep some indoor plants, not only will they remove brain toxic chemicals from your home, their attractive green leafy appearance will lift your spirits.

Chapter Six

The principles for a brain boosting diet and lifestyle

To help you understand why it's important to feed and water your brain correctly here are a few astounding facts

The brain is the fattiest organ in your body, indeed its content is more than 60% fat – so if you call your best friend "fat head", you are giving them a compliment!

75% of the weight of the brain is water – so if you don't drink enough water, don't expect your brain to work well!

There are around 100,000 miles of blood vessels in your brain – so you need to look after your blood vessels!

There are around 100 billion neurones in your brain – that's a lot! Consider that the world's population is 6.5 billion – no wonder you are so smart!

Each neurone has between 1000 to 10,000 connections to other neurones – wow that leaves the internet for dead!

Cholesterol is a vital fat for your brain and it insulates the nerve pathways – if your brain is low in cholesterol it will function more slowly – like dial up internet and not like high speed broadband.

Protein

Every single neurotransmitter in the brain is made of protein. Make sure you have at least three meals daily containing first class protein. They do not have to be large meals or large amounts of protein, but they need to supply the amino acids that the brain requires. Amino acids are the building blocks of protein and they are found in protein foods. The brain's neurotransmitters are made from amino acids.

All the amino acids essential to the manufacture of neurotransmitters are found in first class protein foods such as –

- •Animal protein from foods such as eggs, poultry, dairy products, white and red meats, and seafood
- •Plant protein if it is combined correctly can satisfy the brain's requirements for amino acids. You must combine 3 of the following four food groups at one meal to get all of the amino acids essential for the production of the happy chemicals required by the brain – namely legumes, nuts, seeds and grains. Legumes consist of beans, chickpeas or lentils.

Eating protein regularly prevents large fluctuations in blood sugar levels (hypoglycaemia) and this has a stabilising effect on the mood and mental energy levels.

Reduce sugar and foods high in refined sugar

Foods and beverages, such as chocolate, lollies, cakes, donuts and soft drinks, that contain large amounts of sugar should be decreased and used as occasional treats rather than regular dietary items. Too much sugar will destabilise the blood sugar levels and when the blood sugar levels drop too low, unpleasant mood changes can occur such as anxiety or depression.

Large amounts of sugar can increase the heart rate and cause agitation and hyper stimulation of the nervous system. It is important to avoid large amounts of sugary foods before bedtime as they may cause insomnia. If you need a bed time snack try a protein food such as a piece of cheese or nuts.

Many people feel much calmer and more energetic when they reduce sugary foods and increase dietary protein.

Avoid the artificial sweetener aspartame, which is found in many diet foods and diet sodas. It is represented on labels by the food additive number 951. Aspartame is an excito-toxin that can seriously disturb function of your brain cells – for more information see www.dorway.com

Increase antioxidant foods

The brain has a high requirement for antioxidants because it is a fatty organ and as such is fragile and prone to oxidative damage from free radicals. Free radicals can attack the brain cells (neurones) causing inflammation and if this is allowed to become chronic, damage to the neurones can occur. This could reduce the ability of neurones to manufacture neurotransmitters and damage the cell membranes of the neurones, interfering with their ability to transmit messages between each other. This can result in mood changes and sluggish mental function.

Free radicals are produced in the body from stress, cigarette smoking, excess alcohol, toxic chemicals, infections and pollution.

Antioxidants neutralise free radicals thereby preventing them from inflicting damage upon brain cells. When a person is under increased stress they use up antioxidants at a faster rate and they need to be replenished on a regular basis.

The most important antioxidants to protect our brain cells are

Vitamin E – found in fresh wheat germ, whole grain cereals, eggs, leafy greens, avocados, raw fresh nuts

Vitamin C – found in citrus fruits, berries, kiwi fruits and many other fresh fruits

Selenium – because of soil deficiencies and mass produced food (including farmed fish) it is hard to get enough selenium in your food; so a supplement of 100 mcg daily is advisable. Dietary sources of selenium include broccoli, mushrooms, cabbage, onions, garlic, radishes, brewer's yeast, fish and organ meats.

Phyto-chemicals are powerful antioxidants found in fresh fruits and vegetables. They include sulphur containing chemicals (such as glucosinolates and isothiocyanates), chlorophyll, anthocyanidins and many more. The pigments which give fruits and vegetables their bright colours are also powerful antioxidants. Try to eat one large vegetable salad containing five different colours of vegetables daily. Also aim to eat two pieces of fresh fruit daily. Choose fruits that are in season.

Cold pressed oils such as olive oil, avocado oil, and macadamia nut oil make the salads tasty and provide beneficial fats for the brain.

Fresh green herbs – these are very high in antioxidants and magnesium and can be used in salads or juices. It can be quite therapeutic and also fun to start a little herb garden at home to grow your own organic herbs. I suggest you grow the following – parsley, mint, basil, coriander, thyme, rosemary, shallots and garlic chives. Mint is excellent for lifting the spirits and cleansing the system. Thyme is an excellent natural antibiotic and garlic chives, coriander and basil are liver tonics.

Eating or juicing fresh herbs and vegetables is important for a healthy liver and improving your liver function can help to overcome depression. Metaphysically speaking, the liver is "the seat of anger" so if your liver is overloaded, overworked or toxic you may feel more angry, irritable and moody. Anger turned inwards can make you depressed and many natural therapists recommend a good detox of the liver and bowels to cleanse the mind of irritant toxins. I think there is great merit in this and improving your liver function by eating more raw fresh fruits, vegetables and herbs often clears the mind as well as improving your spirits. For similar reasons you may find that a good liver tonic improves your moods.

Healthy happy fats for the brain

Depression and anxiety can be greatly aggravated if the diet does not provide adequate amounts of the essential fatty acids. The most important fatty acids for the brain are the omega 3 fatty acids known as EPA and DHA. The body cannot manufacture its own supply of these fatty acids – that is why they are called essential!

Studies have shown that in depressed subjects who have a poor diet devoid or very low in omega 3 fatty acids, a remarkable improvement in mental and emotional health is achieved by giving supplements of fish oil. Scans of the brains of these depressed subjects showed that the size of the brain increased after giving the fish oil supplements and especially the areas of the brain concerned with emotion and memory.

I am not surprised by the findings of these studies, as when one considers what the brain is made of, it is quite logical and not unexpected. If we remove the water content from the human brain we find that approximately 70% of its solid mass is comprised of fat, but not just any old fat! You would not want to have a brain made of margarine or cheap cooking oil! The predominant fat found in the brain is omega 3 fatty acid. There are also large amounts of pure cholesterol found in the healthy human brain. Other fats in the brain are phospholipid fats and omega 6 fatty acids. The brain is the fattiest or oiliest organ in your body and it's meant to be like that.

So if you suffer with depression and/or anxiety or poor cognition, take a look at your diet. Do you regularly eat oily fish such as salmon, sardines, tuna, mackerel, herrings, anchovies etc? If not, then you are probably deficient in the happy omega 3 fats, which could be making you depressed.

For similar reasons I am not a fan of the low fat diet craze, as low fat diets do not supply the brain tissue with enough fat; this can increase the risk of depression, anxiety and dementia. It has been found that very low levels of cholesterol in the blood (less than 4.7 mmol/L) are associated with a higher incidence of depression.

If you do not eat plenty of oily fish, I recommend fish oil supplements, ideally in a liquid form; there are lime and orange flavoured liquid fish oils available. If you hate the taste of fish oil, take the capsules. Generally in depressed people I recommend 2000 to 4000mg of pure high quality fish oil daily. In those with a very poor diet, higher doses of 6000 to 8000 mg daily may be required to lift the depression.

If you keep your fish oil in the fridge and take it just before you eat, it should not cause digestive upset or an unpleasant after taste. I prefer to use the liquid forms of fish oil especially if large doses are required. This is because the large soft gelatin capsules which contain the fish oil may contain substances that induce allergies or digestive upsets when taken in large amounts over long periods of time. My preferred fish oil is high quality and flavoured with lemon/lime oils and found in a glass bottle. This is more expensive and not everyone can afford this, so capsules can be used instead. Krill oil is also a good source of omega 3 fatty acids. Krill are tiny shrimp like crustaceans found in the cold oceans.

If you are intolerant or allergic to fish or fish oil, you can obtain omega 3 fatty acids by taking flaxseed oil in liquid or capsule form. Make sure the flaxseed oil is of high quality and once opened it should be kept in the fridge. Generally 2000 to 4000mg daily of flaxseed oil is required; so check the label to see the amount of liquid or the number of capsules you need to take.

Some folks just hate taking oily supplements and for these people I suggest they boost their intake of omega 3 essential fatty acids by taking one to two tablespoons daily of ground whole flaxseeds. You can buy whole flaxseeds and pass them through a food processor or grinder to produce a tasty sweet flavoured powder. You can also buy the flaxseed powder but make sure it looks fresh. Flaxseed powder should be kept in the fridge because fatty acids are fragile and easily become rancid; once rancid they are useless. I keep my flaxseed powder in the freezer where it stays fresh much longer. Flaxseed powder can be stirred into cereals, yoghurt or smoothies and even children enjoy its sweet nutty taste.

The brain's circulation

Eating oily fish and/or taking fish oil supplements helps to improve the circulation of blood to the brain which improves the supply of oxygen to the brain. Oxygen is required for the production of neurotransmitters. If you are allergic to fish oil, take cold pressed flaxseed oil or ground whole flaxseeds instead, to improve your circulation. Vitamin C is essential for a healthy circulation and strong blood vessels in the body and this is another reason to consume citrus fruits, kiwi fruit, berries and capsicum. Spices such as chilli, cayenne, ginger and turmeric stimulate and improve the circulation and can be invigorating to use in your cooking. Foods such as radishes, garlic, chives and onion help to thin the blood thereby improving the circulation.

Magnesium supplements support a healthy muscle tone in your cerebral arteries and can increase the micro-circulation of oxygen rich blood to the brain cells. If you have high blood pressure it is vital to keep it under control, as sustained excessive blood pressure will damage the brain's circulation and increase the incidence of strokes. By keeping the blood thin with fish oil, oily fish and/or flaxseed oil and the other foods and spices mentioned above, you will greatly improve the circulation of blood to your brain and reduce your risk of strokes.

Regular exercise improves the cardiac output and fitness, improving circulation to the brain.

There are around 100,000 miles of blood vessels in your brain which illustrates how much the brain depends upon a circulation of fresh oxygenated blood to every neurone you have!

Get hydrated

Insufficient intake of water can have many adverse health effects and when it comes to your brain, hydration is vital as around 75% of the brain consists of water. Depressed people often consume a lot of coffee or caffeine containing sweet drinks such as soft drinks. These beverages can be dehydrating and will not take the place of water. Dehydrated brain cells do not perform their functions well and lack of water also makes the blood thicker, reducing the circulation to the brain. Try to drink at least 8 glasses of water daily and ideally around 2 litres of water daily will optimise brain function. Herbal tea can be classed as water but don't use too much sugar as then it becomes dehydrating. Try using stevia or xylitol instead to sweeten your beverages. Increasing your water intake not only improves mental energy and moods but also reduces aches and pains and headaches.

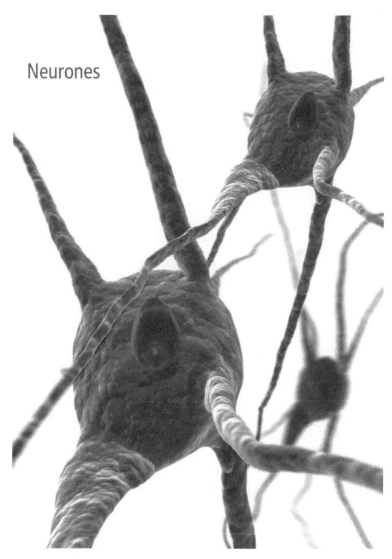

Neurones

High functioning brain cells known as neurones, require large amounts of fats, namely omega 3 fats, phospholipids, and cholesterol to function efficiently. If your brain is deficient in these fats, it will function more slowly and you may become depressed.

Antidepressant Nutrients	Food Sources
Omega 3 fatty acids	Oily fish (salmon, sardines, mackerel, anchovies, tuna, trout, herrings), fish oil, krill oil, flaxseeds, walnuts, green leafy vegetables, organic eggs.
Magnesium	Green leafy vegetables, green leafy herbs, nuts, seeds, molasses, kelp
Zinc	Seafood, miso, red meat, liver, mushrooms, green leafy vegetables
Vitamin D	Sunlight, oily fish, liver, cod liver oil, milk, eggs
Vitamin B 12 (cyanocobalamin)	Meat, seafood, dairy products, organic or free-range eggs, poultry
Vitamin C	Citrus fruits, capsicum, parsley, kiwi fruit, berries, pawpaw, mango, tomato
Vitamin B 3 (niacin)	Poultry, seafood, red meat, liver, tomato, lettuce, mushrooms
Vitamin B 1 (thiamine)	Tuna, peas, eggplant, sunflower seeds, mushrooms, asparagus, spinach, celery
Vitamin B 2 (riboflavin)	Dairy products, eggs, mushroom, liver, asparagus, broccoli, silverbeet

Antidepressant Nutrients	Food Sources
Vitamin B 5 (pantothenic acid)	Eggs, yoghurt, strawberries, tomato, sunflower seeds, liver, mushrooms, broccoli, cauliflower
Vitamin B 6 (pyridoxine)	Mushroom, cabbage, banana, garlic, capsicum, seafood, spinach, cauliflower, asparagus
Folic acid	Green leafy vegetables, cauliflower, asparagus, lentils
Potassium	Molasses, mushrooms, cucumber, squash, fennel, silverbeet, spinach, lettuce, bananas, most fruits
Tryptophan	Seafood, poultry, meat, dairy products, avocados, eggs, wheat germ, banana
Tyrosine	Milk and cheese, poultry, fish, almonds, bananas, red meat and avocados, eggs
Iodine	Seaweed, iodised salt, wild (not farmed) fish
Dopamine and noradrenalin rich foods	Avocados, lima beans, bananas, almonds, pumpkin seeds, sesame seeds, cheese

Herbal teas

If you are drinking excessive amounts of caffeine-containing beverages this may cause anxiety, irritability and poor sleep. As an alternative you could try dandelion coffee, which is good for the liver, and/or herbal teas sweetened with a small amount of honey, stevia or xylitol.

There are specific herbs that have a calming and nurturing effect on the nervous system; these include:

Chamomile, hops, peppermint, lavender flowers, blackberry leaves, wild strawberry leaves, raspberry leaves, rosehips, sunflower blossoms, rose flowers, salvia leaves, lemongrass, orange blossoms, citrus peels and hibiscus.

Pamper yourself

Symptoms of depression often include the loss of enjoyment in the simple things in life and the loss of interest in giving oneself personal pleasure and rewards.

Here are some pampering ideas that may rekindle your senses and help you to relax with yourself.

1. Try a hot bath with one teacup of Epsom salts; this relaxes the muscles and the nerves and lowers the blood pressure. Alternatively use essential oils in your hot bath such as:

Lavender – 3 drops
Ylang Ylang – 3 drops
Basil – 2 drops
Geranium – 2 drops
Grapefruit – 2 drops

Fill the bathtub with hot or warm water, add the essential oils. Close the bathroom door and relax. Light a pretty candle, play your favourite relaxing music, unwind and enjoy!

2. Book yourself in for a deep tissue massage with a therapeutic massage practitioner.

3. Try aromatherapy, as the sense of smell is received and processed in the temporal lobes of the brain and these lobes have direct connections to parts of the brain concerned with strong emotions, past memories and judgment. Several essential oils can slow brain wave patterns to produce sensations of relaxation and calmness. Their method of action is similar to sedative type drugs but much milder.

Suitable oils to put in your diffuser include:

Clary Sage, Marjoram, Neroli, Ylang Ylang, Vetiver, Rose, Lavender, Roman Chamomile, Helichrysum, Lemon, Mandarin, Spikenard and Frankincense.

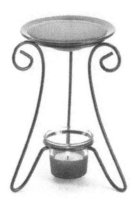

Ask your partner to give you a massage with the following aromatic oil mixture:

Petitgrain – 6 drops
Orange – 5 drops
Neroli – 4 drops
Add the above mixture to 15 ml of almond oil and shake well.

Buy yourself an oil burner (a diffuser) in which you can mix a calming combination of essential oils to burn.

Choose 2 to 3 of the following to burn at one time:

Clary Sage – 10 drops
Lavender – 18 drops
Rosewood– 15 drops
Roman Chamomile – 12 drops
Ylang Ylang – 10 drops
Marjoram – 8 drops
Geranium – 12 drops

Blend into a small glass container and shake well.
Add to your oil burner (diffuser).

A powerful oil mixture to sooth a troubled mind consists of:

4 drops – Lime
4 drops – Sandalwood
6 drops – Bergamot

Blend all the above oils and use in diffuser or place
5–6 drops in your bath.

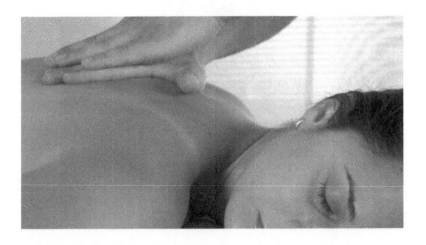

Sleep is essential

Sleep is a safety valve for an over pressured nervous system. If you cannot achieve a deep and restful sleep on a regular basis your nervous system and adrenal gland function will deteriorate. Depression and anxiety are associated with imbalances in neurotransmitters and hormones and these imbalances often cause or exacerbate insomnia. Antidepressant drugs will restore a normal sleep cycle whereas sleeping tablets and sedatives are habituating and should only be used short term. Alcohol excess disrupts the sleep cycle.

I have found that sleep often becomes a problem for women during and after menopause when it is disrupted by hot flushes, overheating of the body and sweating. Sometimes this overheating is due to lack of oestrogen and can be fixed with natural bio-identical hormone replacement creams.

Overheating of the body and disrupted sleep can also be a sign of liver dysfunction especially in those with a poor diet, fatty liver or alcohol dependency. Thankfully we can easily improve the liver function with a liver tonic available over the counter, increasing raw vegetable salads and fruits in the diet and reducing sugar and carbohydrate intake. The most common causes of liver dysfunction are excess dietary sugar, excess alcohol and "polypharmacy" (taking too many prescribed drugs at once). So once again we see the importance of a healthy liver in achieving healthy deep sleep, body temperature control and calm moods.

Melatonin – the sleep hormone

Melatonin is the natural sleep hormone produced in the pea sized gland called the pineal gland. The pineal gland is situated in the middle of your brain. When the eyes are deprived of light the pineal gland is activated to secrete melatonin, which makes you feel sleepy and relaxed. During a normal night's sleep your melatonin levels stay elevated for around 12 hours (usually between 9 pm and 9 am). Artificial lights in the home and from televisions and computers etc reduce the production of melatonin.

Melatonin supplements can be helpful for insomnia and doses range from 1 to 3 mg taken 2 hours before retiring to bed. A doctor's prescription is required for melatonin.

Magnesium supplements can improve sleep and reduce palpitations, muscular tension, nocturnal cramps and restless legs.

Herbal remedies to help sleep include wild lettuce (30 to 120mg before bed), hops (30 to 120mg before bed) and valerian (200 to 800mg before bed).

For more information on sleep problems see the book *"Tired of not sleeping? Holistic remedies for a good night's sleep"*

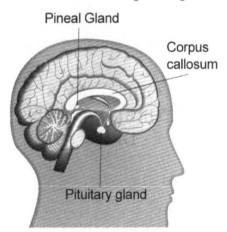

Pineal Gland

Corpus callosum

Pituitary gland

Chapter Seven

Panic Attacks

A panic attack occurs when your level of anxiety and stress becomes intolerable. This stress overload causes your usual defence and coping mechanisms to break down and they are no longer strong enough to keep the anxiety under control. Eventually it comes flooding through into your conscious mind resulting in a panic attack or a state of acute anxiety.

Psychological defence mechanisms were first defined by the famous psychiatrist and neurologist Sigmund Freud. Freud described the way the subconscious mind keeps psychological conflict under control, so that a person can continue to function.

These psychological defence mechanisms included such things as

Suppression –
your mind simply suppresses the conflict and anxiety

Rationalisation –
your mind develops its own logical dialogue as to why things are so bad and these arguments are more acceptable to you than the reality of a situation.

Sublimation –
your mind converts the conflict anxiety into physical symptoms such as headaches, irritable bowel syndrome, muscular aches and pain or other physical problems.

There are more defence mechanisms than this; however these three serve to show you how the subconscious mind and the ego work together to allow a person to function whilst deep seated psychological conflicts exist.

Once the anxiety can no longer be controlled, an acute anxiety state or a panic attack will occur. During a panic attack the body is rapidly flooded with the hormones adrenalin and noradrenalin.

Excess Adrenalin has the following effects

Stimulates and prepares the brain for fight or flight

Speeds up the rate of the heartbeat making the heart and pulse race

Stimulates the rate of breathing

Elevates the blood pressure

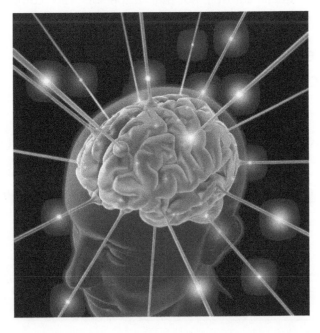

Other possible symptoms during a panic attack include

A thumping sensation inside the chest (but not chest pain)

Extreme weakness of the limbs

Shaking of the limbs

Shortness of breath or air hunger

Pins and needles, tingling and numbness

Involuntary spasm in the hands and feet –
this is called carpopedal spasm

Dizziness and light headedness

Nausea

Intense fear of the unknown

A feeling of impending loss of control and helplessness

A feeling of imminent death

A feeling that some serious medical emergency is about to befall you

If the sufferer of a panic attack is not able to find relief, extreme agitation and collapse may occur. A panic attack is caused by the reaction of the various bodily organs to the effects of excess adrenalin. A panic attack will not cause any serious or significant medical problems and is not caused by a heart attack or lung disease. It is important that a person who is prone to panic attacks, understands what is going on in their body during the attack, otherwise the frightening and unpleasant symptoms of the excess adrenalin often make the panic attack much worse. The sufferer may then have the illusory perception that they are facing a heart attack or imminent death; none of these things will happen during a panic attack.

How to cope with a panic attack

During a panic attack it is important to tell yourself that it is only the excess adrenalin that is making you anxious. Here are some self help techniques to shorten the duration and lower the severity of your symptoms

1. Find a quiet place and lie down and breathe slowly and deeply – stop all thoughts and concentrate on your breath – as you breathe in, feel your energy and strength coming back into you; as you breathe out, feel your stress leaving your body

2. If your heart is beating too fast, there is a technique you can do to slow down the rate of your heartbeat and this is called The Valsalva Manoeuvre (VM). You should not attempt to do the VM without checking with your own doctor first. The VM may not be safe in those who have had a recent heart attack or coronary artery disease. To do the VM, you must lie down first and once lying down take a deep breath and hold it in; then increase the pressure inside your chest by breathing out but don't let any air out. To achieve this keep your lips and nose closed and try to breath or force the air out of your chest. Hold the pressure in your chest until your heart beat slows to a normal and pleasant rate. The VM is a well known technique for slowing the heart beat and is based on physiology. When you do the VM, you increase the pressure inside your chest cavity and this reduces the return of venous blood flow into the heart; this in turn reduces the rate of the heartbeat. You must lie down before doing the VM or it could cause you to faint.

3. Lie down or sit down and slow down the rate of your breathing by counting up to 3 in between each breath. If you breathe too rapidly during a panic attack, you drop the levels of carbon dioxide in your blood stream and this causes the levels of available calcium in your blood to drop rapidly. These low calcium levels can result in involuntary and uncomfortable and even painful spasms in your hands and feet, as well as tingling and numbness in the fingers, toes and around the mouth. Nothing bad or dangerous is happening to your body, it's just that you are breathing too fast.

I think a good analogy to a panic attack is flying through a thunderstorm. I have been a pilot for many years and have flown through quite a bit of bad weather. Pilots are trained to avoid thunderstorms; however sometimes it is necessary to fly in close proximity to them, especially if there is a line of them (this is called a frontal system). The pilot sees the bad weather ahead and prepares to traverse it by slowing down the aircraft, securing loose objects in the cabin and tightening the seat belts. As soon as the dark stormy clouds are penetrated, things start to get very bumpy, and if it's too rough, the adrenalin levels of the pilot will go up slightly. Eventually, usually after 5 to 15 minutes, the aircraft pops out the other side of the stormy clouds into smooth much clearer air; things are then much more comfortable and the pilot relaxes.

Just like stormy clouds, a panic attack does not last forever, and soon you will pop out the other side into a clearer smoother and brighter emotional state. Whilst you are in the "thunderstorm" of the panic attack recognise it is there; yes it is happening, face it, don't try to fight it, but understand that it's only temporary and try to relax inside it. You will pop out the other side – just try the techniques above to relax until it passes. Try to slide or float through it. You will become stronger, just like a pilot who has to learn how to safely traverse bad weather to gain his/her experience, you will become stronger and more in control by learning how to slide through these panic attacks.

Chapter Eight

Hormones and depression

In some types of depression and anxiety, hormonal imbalances play a large causal role. I have seen this countless times over more than 30 years of medical practice and I am often still surprised by the beneficial effect natural hormone therapies can exert upon the emotional and mental state of my patients.

Progesterone –the calm, happy hormone

Progesterone is a sex hormone that is made by the female ovaries during the latter half of the menstrual cycle and in vast amounts during pregnancy. Progesterone exerts a calming effect and can promote contentment and stability. The brain has receptors for many hormones and this is why natural hormones can be so beneficial for emotional disorders.

If you find that your mood lowers during the one to two weeks before your menstrual bleeding commences, then you will probably benefit from natural progesterone. Progesterone deficiency is very common in women today because they often delay pregnancy to later in life and have fewer pregnancies. Progesterone deficiency can cause unpleasant moods such as anxiety, irritability, irrational thinking and depression. Progesterone deficiency can also cause physical health problems such as heavy and/or painful menstrual bleeding, endometriosis, fibroids, increased risk of cancer, premenstrual headaches, polycystic ovarian syndrome and unexplained infertility.

Progesterone deficiency is common in:

Young women with menstrual problems

Women after childbirth where it is associated with postnatal depression

Women after miscarriage

Peri-menopausal women

It is not generally useful to do blood or salivary tests to prove that a deficiency of progesterone exists, as a doctor who understands this hormone can tell from the history of the patient. Keeping a menstrual calendar of symptoms to show your doctor can help to pinpoint the premenstrual exacerbation. For more information see my book *"Don't Let Your Hormones Ruin Your Life"*.

The good news is that natural progesterone therapy can often alleviate these types of hormonal depression in women. Thus one would think that natural progesterone is commonly prescribed for these diverse and common problems. In reality few doctors prescribe natural progesterone because it cannot be patented by drug companies and thus it is not promoted to doctors and doctors are not educated about its use or benefits. This is a pity and results in much unneeded suffering.

The best way to administer natural progesterone is in the form of a cream which is rubbed into the skin of the inner upper arm or the inner upper thigh. The cream can be used once or twice daily and required doses range from 20mg to 400mg daily. You will need a doctor's prescription for natural progesterone and it is made up into a cream by a compounding pharmacist. Natural progesterone is very safe and is usually free of side effects. If excess doses of progesterone are used, the only side effects are bloating, break through bleeding, constipation and feeling too relaxed. In cases of severe premenstrual depression, menopausal depression or postnatal depression, an antidepressant drug may need to be used along with the progesterone.

Postnatal depression

Postnatal depression is a serious form of depression that affects 10 to 16% of women who have children. It is precipitated by hormonal, psychological and lifestyle changes. After the placenta is delivered the level of sex hormones in a woman's body plummets to very low levels and some women are very sensitive to these changes. If breast feeding takes place the hormone production from the ovaries remains switched off, so that low levels of sex hormones persist.

Depression may begin during pregnancy when it is often accompanied by anxiety and thus a more appropriate term may be perinatal depression.

After childbirth, feelings of low mood, tearfulness, fears of being a poor mother and not being able to cope are common and are often temporary, when it is known as the postpartum blues. If these symptoms persist for more than several weeks or are severe, a diagnosis of postpartum depression is likely. If a woman remains depressed after childbirth and is not able to function as a mother, antidepressant medication can be life saving. The patient must be closely supervised and hospitalisation may be required, as there is always a danger that the mother may suffer with compulsions to harm herself or her newborn child. A close family network is vitally important with non judgemental and caring support from family and friends.

Depressed women will often not realise that they are depressed and may focus their negative feelings on the behaviour of the baby – for example they may say things like "if only she would stay asleep" or "if only he would stop crying" or "if only he would drink his bottle". In such cases the mother, especially a first time mother or an older mother, may have expectations that are out of sync with normal baby behaviour. It is important for doctors and family members to listen to these concerns sincerely and not to be dismissive. Some babies are difficult and demanding and a woman may need to be supported, reassured and educated that the postnatal period is a time of sleeplessness, intense need and adaption and simple survival strategies may need to be developed. Feeding the baby, getting adequate food and exercise, as well as grabbing every opportunity for rest and sleep are the important priorities.

Natural progesterone therapy can help to alleviate the depression and can be given along with the antidepressant medication. Progesterone is best given as a cream and doses vary from 20 to 400mg daily.

If fatigue is severe, capsules of DHEA may restore energy and lift the mood often within one week of starting them. Doses of DHEA vary from 10 to 30mg daily.

Generally speaking treatment with natural progesterone and/or DHEA does not interfere with breast feeding and is safe to use until the depression passes; this may take quite a few months.

If fatigue or other physical symptoms are predominant it is important to check for medical problems such as thyroid gland disorders, anaemia, adrenal gland exhaustion, immune diseases and nutritional deficiencies which can be specifically treated. One cannot assume that fatigue is just a symptom of depression.

If the patient decides not to breast feed, other hormones may prove helpful to alleviate postnatal depression. Blood tests can be done to test the levels of testosterone and oestrogen and if these are still low 8 weeks after childbirth, a cream containing natural oestrogen and/or testosterone can be used. Oestrogen and testosterone will restore the libido, as well as improve the mood, and if small doses are used in a cream form, there is no increased risk of blood clots occurring. Oestrogen cannot be used if the woman is breast feeding as it may reduce the milk supply.

Supplements of fish oil, magnesium and iron and B group vitamins can help to alleviate postnatal depression and fatigue.

There should be no rush to withdraw a woman with postnatal depression off her antidepressant medication or hormone therapy, as it is a severe form of depression and it is vital to avoid a recurrence. Although infanticide and suicide are uncommon, it is important to recognise that postnatal depression is the major cause of suicide-related maternal death and the risk of infanticide is highest during the first year of life.

Doctors are careful to differentiate between a depressive illness and postpartum psychosis, which presents within the first few days to weeks after childbirth. Women with postpartum psychosis have strong delusions, hallucinations and are very confused, agitated and hyperactive. During postpartum psychosis both the mother and child are at high risk and hospitalisation and medication are essential to avoid tragic outcomes. Postpartum psychosis is more likely to occur in women who have a family history or past history of bipolar disorder, manic depression or schizophrenia.

If a woman becomes seriously depressed during pregnancy or whilst breast feeding, she will have to decide whether to take antidepressant drugs or not – this can be quite a dilemma. This is because her infant will be exposed to the medication to some degree in these cases. Generally speaking antipsychotic and antidepressant drugs are relatively safe during pregnancy and breast feeding. Safety information has been mainly derived from data bases and not double-blind controlled trials and thus this information has limitations. To understand more about risks of drugs during pregnancy see the website www.motherisk.org.

Use of the SSRI drugs is associated with a slightly higher risk of heart defects and pulmonary hypertension. All antidepressants and antipsychotic drugs are associated with a higher risk of slight prematurity (average 39weeks compared with 40 weeks) and withdrawal symptoms in the infant (sleep disturbances and irritability).

There are risks to the mother and child if the depression is not treated effectively, so all the pros and cons need to be considered by the mother and her partner. Not treating perinatal depression is associated with premature birth, low birth weight, poor nutrition, poor bonding with the baby as well as the slight risk of infanticide and maternal suicide.

Psychological support for perinatal depression

In rural centres – psychologists can be accessed via the Better Outcomes program

Books – Left Holding the Baby by Mary Louise Parkinson

Postnatal Depression – a guide for Australian families by Lisa Fettling

Support Groups for depressed postnatal women (not general mothers' groups which may be alienating)

Couple or family therapy from a psychologist

Group Program – PAIRS (Parent and Infant Relationship Support program)

Circle of Security – this American program can be viewed at www.circleofsecurity.org

www.raisingchildren.net.au – a Federal Government Program

www.nswiop.nsw.edu.au and see their video – titled *Getting to know you* – Institute of Psychiatry

Case history

Jenny had been trying for 6 months to have her first child and was using a cream containing natural progesterone to improve her fertility, reduce period pain and make her cycle more regular. The progesterone worked well and after 3 months Jenny was pregnant. Unfortunately she miscarried 12 weeks into her pregnancy and there were some retained products left behind in her uterus which got infected necessitating the use of strong antibiotics. Jenny had an allergic reaction to the antibiotics and 8 weeks after the miscarriage she became emotionally unwell. Jenny had stopped the progesterone cream when she miscarried.

I saw Jenny 12 weeks after her miscarriage. She was highly anxious, hypochondriacal, indecisive, depressed and fatigued and thought that she had been most unfortunate to miscarry. I explained to Jenny that around 25% of pregnancies will miscarry and that a miscarriage is a relatively normal event and that her future chances of a successful pregnancy were very good. Despite my reassurances and extended counselling sessions with her, she remained depressed and anxious and was not coping.

We decided that a short course of antidepressants may be needed; however she asked me if we could try natural progesterone first. I said sure, as it is a very safe treatment and should help her to conceive when she felt ready again.

Two months later Jenny returned to my clinic and her demeanour was completely different. She was no longer depressed, confused or anxious and she did not need counselling. Rather Jenny spent the next half hour telling me how miraculous natural progesterone was! In her case, her choice not to take antidepressant drugs had worked. Once again, as many times before, here was a young woman reminding me about the restorative and calming power of natural progesterone.

Testosterone – the confident sexy hormone

Testosterone is the male hormone and is made in large amounts by the testicles and in smaller amounts in women by the ovaries. A deficiency of testosterone is more likely to cause a depressive or anxiety type illness in men, especially once they get to middle age or beyond. Men who are overweight or diabetic are more likely to have a testosterone deficiency. Marijuana use, especially if chronic, greatly reduces the amount of testosterone in the blood.

There are receptors in the brain for testosterone and the effect of testosterone is to make a person feel more assertive, aggressive, confident, energetic and sexy.

Blood tests should be done to determine if there is a testosterone deficiency present and the normal ranges vary from women to men. Blood tests are highly accurate and much cheaper and more reliable than salivary hormone testing.

It is important to check the blood levels of the total and the free testosterone because it is only the free testosterone that is available to your brain.

Natural testosterone can be prescribed by your doctor in the form of a gel or cream and the doses vary depending upon how low your own blood levels of testosterone are. It is safer, and just as effective, to take testosterone as a skin cream or gel than it is to take a tablet or injection of testosterone.

Most doctors are aware of the beneficial effect that testosterone therapy can have in people who have low blood testosterone levels and who suffer with depression, anxiety, fatigue, withdrawal, loss of confidence or loss of libido.

DHEA –the resilience and endurance hormone

The hormone called DHEA (dehydroepiandrosterone) is made in the adrenal glands; as we age, we gradually produce less and less DHEA. If a depressive and/or anxiety type illness is associated with chronic fatigue, especially in the morning, it is important to do a blood test to check the levels of DHEA. In persons over 60 we can expect DHEA levels to be low, but still within the normal range for their age group. Some people who suffer depression and chronic fatigue find that supplements of the hormone DHEA really help them a lot, especially in the area of feeling more energetic and more emotionally stable. Perhaps this is because DHEA exerts a mild testosterone and steroid like effect.

DHEA can be equally effective for men and women who have chronic fatigue associated with depression and anxiety.

In people who have been exposed to severe or long term stress, DHEA supplements can greatly help to overcome the symptoms of adrenal gland exhaustion.

DHEA can be administered as a cream, capsule or lozenge and doses vary from 10mg to 50mg daily. There are no known side effects of DHEA, although in some people high doses can promote acne and weight gain. Always start with a low dose and see if that works; if needed, the dose can be increased.

Not all doctors are aware of the benefits of DHEA in emotional illness and/or chronic fatigue, but if you have a compounding pharmacist in your area, ask them if there is a local doctor who prescribes it.

Homoeopathic versions of DHEA, or for that matter other hormones, are generally not effective. To get effective doses of natural hormones, a doctor's prescription is required.

Testimonial

I crashed badly in late 2007, after a full hysterectomy and major surgery to remove a 20cm uterine tumour. I was told the surgery was a success, but twelve months later I didn't feel much better. The hot flushes and long hot night sweats that started up immediately after surgery were still there.

Hormone replacement therapy didn't seem to help – in any case it gave me headaches. I had chronic fatigue that was a bit like the flu and I slept most of the day. My house with all its mess and piled up dishes started to look like a candidate for a TV current affairs story. I couldn't care for my children properly – dinner was McDonalds 4 times a week or whatever they found themselves in the cupboards.

My gut seemed to erode itself away for unknown reasons, and that would make me extremely sick. I took activated charcoal to clear out the nausea every morning and I spent my day in pain and with a strange nasty sort of physical discomfort that was unbearable.

I was too sick to work, and I was spending a hundred dollars a week from my Centrelink welfare payment for supplements just to keep myself in my current state of sickness. I was particularly upset that I would probably have to drop my law degree. As a single welfare mother, I had worked extremely hard to get there. I was just hanging in there with the aid of strong stimulants to get me through each exam or assignment. I had developed severe ADHD and without them, I could not focus and would fall asleep. The constant stimulants were making me sick but I didn't know any other way. Doctors could offer me nothing except blood tests which all came back normal.

Out of desperation I started buying Dr Sandra Cabot's self help books. Actually, I purchased just about every self help book from every bookstore in Adelaide. Amongst other things I learnt from Dr Cabot's book that a dysfunctional liver was connected to numerous significant health problems, and the dysfunction didn't necessarily show up in conventional diagnostic tests.

Inside Cabot's book titled *The Liver Cleansing Diet* was an 8 week program which was simple and inexpensive, using nutritional whole foods. It was financially viable for a pensioner to follow. For me it offered the only prospect of recovery from any source. The program required following a simple eating plan, using the recipes provided. There was plenty of choice, with the worst part of the program involving trying to get down eight glasses of water a day, especially when it had lemon in it.

In 2008, before starting the diet, I received a $2000 payment as part of the Rudd government's economic stimulus policy. I resolved to stimulate the economy by flying to Sydney (from Adelaide) for an appointment with Dr Cabot in person. I felt sufficiently sick and dysfunctional to require additional help. I couldn't imagine what she could do for me but I felt quite desperate.

I was shocked when Dr Cabot informed me that I had a depressive illness – or at least I would have been shocked if I had had the energy. I'm not sure I really believed her. She also diagnosed some hormone imbalances that other doctors would not have picked up from the test results. I was given DHEA, which regulates a number of hormones, plus her own thyroid preparation. There were also raw juice instructions and digestive enzymes, as I wasn't digesting anything properly.

I arrived back in Adelaide and took the hormones. Within a week, my pain had been cut in half and the sweats and flushes dissolved into almost nothing. In addition, I just felt better. I read up on the antidepressant Dr Cabot prescribed for me. It was called Parnate and was described as very strong preparation given for quite severe cases of depression, and designed to give relief within 48 hours. Again I was stunned. Somewhat apprehensive I bit the bullet and started to take it.

I started feeling the effects within hours. By the end of the week I was all but out of pain, and the strange nasty physical discomfort had all but vanished. I can't describe the relief. It reminded me of being in labour and finally getting the baby out. I was physically comfortable and that changed my whole quality of life.

Dr Cabot then sent me an email in capital letters reminding me that I HAD to treat my liver. I was physically comfortable, somewhat more functional, and now had enough energy to make a start on the Liver Cleansing Diet. Her 'L shaped' homoeopathic formula stopped the cravings for junk and I discovered that smoothies made with her Syndrome X protein powder and frozen raspberries were really yummy. Hummus, tomato and cucumber on Corn Thins was delicious. I still don't know how to cook brown rice.

About three days into the diet, I noticed that I didn't wake up every morning with nausea. I didn't have to clear out toxins which must have been generated from my previous diet. That's $13 a week I didn't have to spend on charcoal. Then I realized I didn't have to use my gut repair powder. My gut didn't seem to be eroding anymore. That was a further $40 a week I didn't have to spend.

The brain fog started to clear up, and I received my first distinction grade for a Law essay and managed to complete my 3000 word research paper 2 weeks later. I don't fall asleep during the day anymore. I can get my housework done and my kids get proper meals on the table – the same as I have on the Liver Cleansing Diet. They are less appreciative of Dr Cabot's efforts than I am however – they prefer Big Macs and double chocolate sundaes for dinner.

By Mrs Hayes, Adelaide South Australia

Adrenal gland exhaustion

The adrenal glands are often called "the survival glands" because they manufacture powerful energising hormones and messenger chemicals such as adrenalin, DHEA cortisol, and other steroid hormones.

In people who have been under prolonged physical and/or mental stress the adrenal glands can become depleted resulting in chronic and debilitating fatigue. The condition of adrenal gland exhaustion can result in a stress breakdown where a person is unable to function. Other symptoms of adrenal gland exhaustion include low blood pressure, dizziness, fainting attacks, excess inflammation and inability to cope with normal levels of stress.

Adrenal gland exhaustion is not the same condition as adrenal gland failure (which is known as Addison's disease). In adrenal gland exhaustion, blood tests of adrenal gland function are usually within the normal ranges, although often the blood levels of cortisol and DHEA are at the lower limits of the normal range. In Addison's disease blood tests will be grossly abnormal.

Your local doctor can test your adrenal glands by measuring blood cortisol levels in the morning and late afternoon, by doing a 24 hour urine collection to measure the amount of cortisol excreted in the urine over a 24 hour period, and blood DHEA levels.

I treat cases of adrenal gland exhaustion with supplements of fish oil, vitamin C, selenium and magnesium. It is often highly beneficial to include some prescription DHEA from a compounding chemist. Doses of DHEA vary from 20 to 50mg daily depending upon body weight, age, sex and the severity of the exhaustion. DHEA is best prescribed as capsules.

It is also important to get more rest and relaxation in such cases.

Menopause and depression

Over many years of practising medicine I have found that menopause is a common time for women to find themselves going through new, strange and often unpleasant emotions and these can include:

Depression

Anxiety

Insomnia, often exacerbated by hot flushes

Loss of confidence

Loss of libido

Loss of interest

This is often brought on by the following factors

The stress of having to care for elderly and unwell aged parents

The empty nest syndrome caused by children leaving the home environment

The loss of sex hormones – oestrogen, progesterone and testosterone

Menopause is a time when the subconscious mind often becomes more active and strong and primitive emotions can breakthrough into the conscious mind. For example you have reached a phase of your life where you have worked hard for years, raised children and cared for others. You start thinking of the things you want to achieve for yourself on a personal level but may be frustrated by lack of time or resources and the fact that you are getting older.

The subconscious mind harbours our deeper desires for satisfaction, getting back to the meaning of life, freedom and pleasure. Menopause can be a wonderful and potentially liberating time of life, if we feel physically and mentally well; it is a great opportunity to undertake new ventures to develop a foundation for middle age and old age.

I encourage peri-menopausal women to undertake new courses and hobbies to improve their intellectual capabilities and to start taking the time for themselves to fulfil their dreams and passions. Exercise is even more important as you get older and has many advantages including increased energy, less depression, less fatigue, improved cardiovascular health and less risk of osteoporosis.

Some women find that natural bio-identical hormone replacement in the form of creams can relieve their symptoms and improve their sex life as well as their physical relationships.

Blood tests to check all your hormones are essential and I like to measure the following:

FSH and oestrogen levels

Free testosterone levels

DHEA levels

Thyroid hormones

Keep yourself strong physically and mentally and you will enjoy menopause as a new phase of your life. One of my patients said to me that she was anxious about menopause because her mother had become very depressed soon after menopause and had to be frequently admitted to a mental hospital and receive electric shock therapy. I reassured her that in this day and age the treatments available, including natural hormone therapies and antidepressant drugs, would be able to save her from such an awful experience. During the 1970s we did not have natural hormone therapy or really effective antidepressant drugs and that is why her poor mother had suffered so much.

I have another patient aged 68, who still takes lozenges of natural testosterone and DHEA because these hormones give her mental and physical energy. She finds that she needs these hormones to keep her interest in life going and especially her gardening, as she is a keen gardener with a beautiful garden. She finds that without the testosterone she loses interest in everything. She does not need any oestrogen or progesterone, as she is not in an active sexual relationship. We are all very different and that is why it is important to individualise treatment for peri-menopausal and post menopausal women.

Thyroid hormone and depression

Lack of thyroid hormone can cause depression and poor memory. In depressed patients who also complain of fatigue, poor memory, elevated cholesterol and difficulty losing weight it is vital to do a blood test to check the function of the thyroid gland. The condition of low or under active thyroid gland function is quite common and treatment is often delayed, which is a pity, as if we optimise thyroid gland function we can get a remarkable improvement in mood, cognition and energy levels. If blood tests reveal a clearly under active thyroid gland it is easy to relieve the symptoms of this by giving thyroid hormone tablets or capsules. Some patients respond better by taking both types of thyroid hormone (namely Oroxine and Tertroxin).

If a person is low in the minerals selenium and iodine (and these deficiencies are very common), the function of their thyroid gland and their thyroid metabolism will be sluggish; this can cause fatigue, mental slowness and moodiness.

Thyroid health capsules are designed to provide adequate amounts of iodine, selenium and vitamin D for optimal thyroid function. Thyroid health capsules are available from health food stores and/or pharmacies and do not require a prescription.

An overactive thyroid gland can cause the symptoms of anxiety – namely tremor, racing heart beat, palpitations, diarrhoea, weight loss and agitation. Once again it's important to check the thyroid gland function with a simple blood test.

For more in-depth information on the holistic treatment of thyroid problems, see my book "Your Thyroid Problems Solved" or visit www.aboutthyroid.com or call the Health Advisory Service on (02) 4655 8855.

Vitamin D – the sunshine hormone

Many researchers think of vitamin D as a hormone rather than a simple vitamin. I agree with this because vitamin D does exert hormone like actions in the brain and skeleton. Vitamin D is made from cholesterol in the skin. When the sun's ultraviolet B (UVB) rays penetrate the exposed skin the cholesterol is turned into vitamin D. Vitamin D is required for a healthy nervous system and a healthy immune system.

The lack of vitamin D during the winter months may explain the type of depression that only affects people during the seasons when less sunshine is available – this type of depression is called "seasonal affective disorder".

In depressed persons who avoid sunshine, it is important to check the blood levels of vitamin D; if these are found to be low, this could be exacerbating depression, fatigue and aches and pains (fibromyalgia).

You would think that most people living in sunny climates produce plenty of vitamin D but I have found that over 50% of my patients have low or suboptimal levels of vitamin D in their blood. This is because people work long hours indoors and when outside, they cover up and use sunscreen, which blocks vitamin D production in the skin. So if you are depressed and low in vitamin D you should spend some time relaxing in the sun with your clothes off. As a guide, Dr Craig Hassed who is senior lecturer at Monash University's Department of General Practice, recommends you need 10–15 minutes of sunshine daily if most of your skin is exposed and the UV index is 7. If the UV index is 3 and you have more clothes on you will need 25 minutes in the sun. If you are older or of dark complexion you will need more time in the sun. Avoid the midday sun in the middle of summer to prevent sun burn. It is wise to expose more skin to sunshine and take a vitamin D supplement if your levels are low and you may find that your mental health improves.

Chapter Eight

A plan to become the best you can be

Cognitive and behavioural therapy

L earning how to think and behave in a productive way takes time, practise and discipline. Negative thinking will create negative emotions, so if we learn to counteract negative thoughts with rational and/or positive thoughts, we may avoid the sad and anxious emotions.

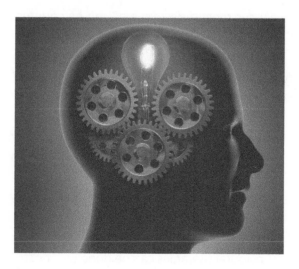

We can learn to question our negative thoughts, for example

"I won't enjoy this" can be answered with *"How do you know, are you a psychic? You will never know if you don't try it"*

"I can't get out of this situation" can be answered with
"Have I considered all my options?"

"I have made a mess of this" can be answered with
"I am not perfect but I am willing to try again"

"I am too tired to exercise" can be answered with
"If I try a little exercise it will give me more energy"

"I am feeling too sad to do anything" can be countered with
"I will start doing something easy and stop thinking"

"I have a right to be negative and angry" can be countered
with *"My attitude will change to one of gratitude for the
good things that are available to me"*

"I am going to fail, as this is beyond me" can be countered
with *"I am going to relax and then think about this step
by step"*

"Everyone always tries to destroy me" can be countered with
*"my detractors must be very bored to have to comment or
focus on me"*

*My mother often quotes Oscar Wilde, who said
"There is only one thing worse than being talked about,
and that is not being talked about"*

"I am so poor, I have lost all my assets" can be countered
with *"my health is the important thing along with my true
friends and I can still enjoy the simple pleasures of life"*

*"The things I plan never work out, so I am a failure
"* can be countered with *"perhaps destiny has a greater
plan for me, which will bring more happiness"*

Cognitive behavioural therapies can be done by a doctor trained
in this area, or a clinical psychologist.

Case history

Mary had found that she was plagued by anxiety and panic attacks, which started in her early 20s. She had often felt disturbed emotionally during childhood.

Mary did find that a low dose of the SSRI drug Aropax helped her to cope because it reduced her anxiety and nightmares and made her more confident. However she told me that it was her use of positive thought and a positive attitude that had helped her to grow in her life and maintain a part time job. Mary was also very spiritual and had close relationships with people at her local church.

Mary had developed successful behavioural strategies and positive thought patterns that she used repetitively in her life. She told me that these included–

Talking to her close friends and family members

Going to church regularly

Putting a smile on her face, even if she felt down and grumpy

Dressing in bright coloured clothes and jewellery

Going to dancing classes and musical concerts

Disallowing negative thoughts, as she knew that negative thoughts produced negative feelings

Telling herself that her mind played tricks and what she was told by her mind was often wrong and did not exist

Writing down positive and inspiring things in her diary

Thinking of others in need and helping out – she called it "getting off yourself"

Forgiving herself and telling herself that she is free from fear

Mary had found that after a panic attack she would often have residual awful and weird feelings in her body for a few days such as butterflies, unsettling sensations, depersonalisation and feelings of losing control – she taught herself to physically wiggle her body to get rid of these feelings and it worked; she would also read the beautiful words in the 23rd psalm.

Mary told me that she never wanted to go back into the awful anxiety and panic states of the past and that is why she had developed her coping strategies over a long period of experimenting to find out which ones worked. She said – it works and I now have power over my mind!

Are you seeking a calm, clear and contented mind?

Well one would think that every person desires to be able to experience a calm, natural and contented state of mind. I know I do.

Ask yourself a few questions:

> Do you ever wish you could still your mind and stop the thoughts that worry, depress or distract you?
>
> Do you ever feel empty and dissatisfied and wonder how to find contentment?
>
> Do you ever feel like a leaf blown helplessly by the wind and think how can I find my anchor?
>
> Do you ever feel like you have lost your power and crave to find an inner power or strength?
>
> Do you spend too much time thinking about the past and the future in a negative way?
>
> Do you find it hard to let go of the past and to live in the present moment like you could when you were a child?

If so there are techniques that can help you to become more in control of your energy and your thoughts and thus your emotions.

The great saints and yogis of history have pursued this quest and they have developed various techniques such as physical yoga, silence, chanting a mantra, prayer, renouncing the world and countless other methods to try and calm the mind. This can seem very difficult to do and perhaps not too appealing! I can imagine that even the greatest yogi sitting on the top of a mountain far away from the conflicts of the world still has difficult days where it rains, the mosquitoes bite and boredom sets in.

Recently I received a brochure in the mail inviting me to a conference called "Happiness and its causes" which I must admit is a cute title! The speakers were internationally famous and included psychologists, psychiatrists, creative thinkers, motivational experts, relationship experts, philanthropists and theologians, ministers of various faiths, sociologists, business experts, human behaviour experts, nutritionists, journalists, philosophers, professors, laughter therapists, futurists and meditation teachers. This conference has been hugely successful over a 3 year period and is the largest conference of its kind in the world. I am sure that this conference would be fascinating and full of new and inspiring ideas. However it is not accessible for everyone, as it is quite expensive and requires travel to Sydney. It would be wonderful to see it recorded and posted on www.youtube.com for all to enjoy, however it is not!

I have found that when one gets a group of experts together, and at this conference there will be more than 50 experts, it can get quite confusing. This is because if you ask 10 different experts a question they often give you 10 different perspectives. You could come away from such a conference with so many ideas and concepts that you feel overloaded.

As we get older we all develop our own unique perspective and ideas and this is what makes people so interesting. The one thing that seems to be universal amongst human beings is that they seek to find happiness – as seen by the success of this conference on happiness.

In reality happiness is a state of mind – it is an experience and is not an idea or concept. I have found that people, including myself, seek to experience a calm, self sufficient, contented state of mind. Sometimes I crave this as strongly as I crave food when I am very hungry or water when I am parched. Contentment seems to be a basic human need and yet many of us find it difficult to stop the thoughts and feelings that get in the way. Negative thoughts and emotions are very powerful and prevent us from living in the present moment – they literally steal away our precious time.

There are techniques we can learn and practise to concentrate our awareness on the powerful and yet peaceful energy that exists within us and sustains our existence. These techniques focus the mind on this beautiful energy, and the thoughts that worry us diminish and gradually go away. I relish doing these techniques because they give me more control over my thoughts and emotions and I enjoy the experience of the powerful and calm energy inside me. I also find that being able to tune into my inner energy makes me feel more confident in myself.

For more information on these techniques see the

website www.wordsofpeace.org

"What lies behind us and what lies before us are small matters compared to what lies within us."

Ralph Waldo Emerson

Create your own plan

If you struggle with emotional illness it is important to develop a plan of action and be armed with foresight gained from the experience and help of others

Here is a suggested plan that you could use as a framework to develop a personal plan for yourself

- If you are not emotionally or mentally well, get help early.

- Avoid using alcohol or self medicating with recreational drugs or over the counter drugs.

- Find a good local doctor and/or a counsellor you can relate to and feel comfortable with and see them regularly. You may need the help of several health care professionals and your local doctor can set up a mental health care plan for you. If you are a full time carer or have postnatal depression you will need the help of a social worker from a public hospital as well as your family.

- Keep your plan simple, as too many ideas on how to get well may confuse and/or overload you – find one approach that works for you, as it can act as a splint for your broken emotions and splintered mind.

- If you are in an intensely stressful situation at work or at home you may need a change of scene, a rest in hospital or a holiday or take some sick leave. If you feel like you need a new environment, accept a change of environment if offered.

- Understand that emotional illness is temporary. If old fears return, remember my analogy of the thunderstorm – don't panic, relax and fly on through it, as there will be clear smooth sunny skies at the other end of the storm. With practise you will get better at this and become a more confident person. Confidence that comes from within you is real and lasting confidence.

- Don't force your recovery and if you are tired, rest and accept your fatigue, as it may take several months to recover.

• Delay major decisions until you have recovered from depression, as your judgment will be clouded by mental confusion, temporary loss of confidence and overload; wait until your old and stronger self returns before making major life changing decisions. You may feel weak and drained now, but once you are recovered you will once again be able to achieve your goals.

• Have a planned program of activities to occupy you or distract you. Do not be bluffed by your thoughts! Remember your greatest enemy is between your ears. If your mind is invaded with painful and fearful thoughts, you need to practise ignoring them. Instead do activities such as exercise, taking a shower or a bath, making some healthy food, read a book, listen to cheerful music or the radio, watch a funny movie or phone your best friend – this type of occupational therapy can distract you from your negative thoughts and emotions until they pass. Occupations such as hobbies, socialising, work or exercise can be a wonderful mental crutch.

• Make sure you have a good physical check up with your doctor or a specialist physician to exclude medical causes of emotional illness and cognitive decline such as:

> Nutritional deficiencies
>
> Anaemia
>
> Brain toxicity from heavy metals
>
> Brain toxicity from environmental chemicals such as cleaning agents, industrial chemicals, insecticides, pesticides etc
>
> Thyroid gland disorders
>
> Deficiencies of hormones such as progesterone, testosterone or DHEA
>
> Blood sugar problems or undiagnosed diabetes
>
> Very high blood pressure
>
> Autoimmune diseases that can affect the brain such as lupus or multiple sclerosis
>
> Disorders of the brain such as brain tumours, dementia, or Parkinson's disease

Infection of the brain with a virus or bacteria

If you have headaches that cannot be controlled ask your doctor for a referral to see a neurologist.

• If you have a mild depression, try using natural antidepressants (see chapter 5); however discuss this with your own doctor or naturopath first. Natural antidepressants have a more subtle effect in relieving emotional disorders and they may take up to 2 to 4 months to really improve the function of your nervous system.

• Trust your own doctor because if you need to take antidepressant drugs, your doctor is trained to recognise this. The most important thing is to get well and not to worry about how you get well.

• Be patient, as some antidepressant drugs take up to 6 weeks to exert their effect and you need to be regular in taking your medication. There is not much you can do until we get your brain chemistry right!

• Have a positive attitude. Understand that depression and anxiety are due to a chemical imbalance, which can be greatly improved and often overcome, no matter how severe the imbalance.

• Be philosophical and wise – understand that happiness can be found within you and don't give up the search, as it is closer than you think. Remember that other people cannot make you happy, so try to lose this expectation. The people you love and are closest to, may be unhappy or confused themselves and not in control of their own emotions or behaviour. You cannot change others; you can only change your attitude. As my grandmother always said "leopards don't change their spots." It is wiser to have expectations only of yourself; this brings detachment and peace and can even give you a sense of liberation. Others can only give you what they are capable of giving and this is often a big variable!

• Don't let guilt make your recovery unpleasant, as you deserve to have your own space and time to recover. Allow yourself the time to get extra sleep, relaxation, exercise and make healthy food and raw juices. Give yourself time, as time is often a great healer in itself. Stop the guilt trip, as this emotion takes away the energy you need to recover! If you believe that you have let yourself or others down, you may experience excessive guilt, which can prevent your recovery. Learn to let go of guilt, as it feeds on itself and fosters depression. You can always make up for your shortfalls when you recover, so practise letting go of the guilt. Give yourself another chance!

I hope this book has given you greater understanding of your mind and emotions and given you some inspiration and direction. There is always hope to find happiness and mental balance and although modern medicine cannot always cure mental and emotional illness, it has advanced in huge strides since the middle of the last century.

Holistic medicine which is caring and considers the mind, body and spirit is the best approach and thankfully there is no longer a stigma around mental and emotional disorders. It is always important to get help early and to reach out to doctors, family and friends. There are excellent books, organisations and Internet resources to help those battling with emotional illness – see page 117–128

Online Resources

Mental Health Links

Mental Health/Psychiatry Internet Resources

http://library.adelaide.edu.auguide/med/mentalhealth/

An extensive list of links maintained by the University of Adelaide Library

Mental Health Branch of the Australian Health Department

http://www.health.gov.au/hsdd/methalhe/

Links to documents such as the National Mental Health Strategy and the

Mental Health Promotion and Prevention National Action Plan

Australian Network for Promotion, Prevention and Early Intervention For Mental Health

http://www.auseinet.com/

Australian network for promotion, prevention and early intervention for mental health, and suicide prevention

The Centre for Rural and Remote Mental Health

http://www.crrmh.com.au/

Mental Health Association NSW Inc

http://www.mentalhealth.asn.au/index.htm

The Mental Health Association NSW Inc is a non-government organization funded by Northern Sydney Area Health. The Association's major activities include provision of the Mental Health Information Service, support groups (including training and establishment of new groups), mental health promotion and advocacy.

SANE Australia

http://www.sane.org/

SANE Australia is a national charity helping people affected by mental illness. The website contains general information about a wide range of mental illness.

Multicultural Mental Health Australia

http://www.mmha.org.au/

Mental health information translated into many languages – also links to culturally-relevant disorders on the causes and symptoms of these disorders, as well as types of treatments and support services are available

Reach Out!

http:www.reachout.com.au

Reach Out! Is a service that uses the Internet to help young people get through tough times. Developed in response to Australia's unacceptably high rates of youth suicide and attempted suicide, Reach Out! Provides much-needed information, assistance and referrals in a format that appeals to young people.

Ethnic Mental Health Program (Australia)

http://ariel.ucs.unimelb.edu.au/%7eatmhn/www.members/emhp.html

The Ethnic Mental Health Program came into being to meet the identified mental health needs of non-English speaking background people. Currently the Program operates in the Chinese, Greek, Italian, Spanish-speaking and Vietnamese Communities in the greater Brisbane area.

Mental Health Research Institute (Aust)

http://www.mhri.edu.au/

The Mental Health Research Institute's mission is to further knowledge in mental health, behaviour and neuroscience. Researchers work to investigate the nature, origins and causes of psychiatric diseases and apply the knowledge they gain to improve diagnosis, treatment and, ultimately, prevent mental illnesses such as Alzheimer's disease and schizophrenia.

National Association of Practising Psychiatrists (Aust)

http://www.ozemail.com.au/~napp/index.html

National Standards for Mental Health Services (Aust)

http://www.health.gov.au/hsdd/mentalhe/nmhs/stand/intro.htm

The project to develop the national standards for mental health services was funded by the Commonwealth Department of Health and Family Services (CDHFS) through the Australian Health Ministers Advisory Council's (AHMAC) National Mental Health Policy Working Group (NMHPWG) as part of the National Mental Health Strategy.

Royal Australian and New Zealand College of Psychiatrists

http://www.ranzcp.org/

Australian Drug Foundation

http://www.adf.org.au

CEIDA Centre for Education and Information on Drugs and Alcohol (Australia)
http://www.ceida.net.au

Narcotics Anonymous Australia

http://www.naoz.org.au/index.htm

Child and Adolescent Mental Health

Australian Early Intervention Network for Mental Health in Young People

http://www.auseinet.com/

Early Psychosis Prevention and Intervention Centre (Aust)

http://www.eppic.org.au/

The Early Psychosis Prevention and Intervention Centre (EPPIC) is a program of North Western Health. The Centre is an integrated and comprehensive psychiatric service aimed at addressing the needs of older adolescents and young adults with emerging psychotic disorders in the western metropolitan region of Melbourne, Australia.

Depression

Blue Pages

http://bluepages.anu.edu.au/

BluePages provides information about depression for consumers. It is produced by the Centre for Mental Health Research at the Australian National University and CSIRO Mathematical & Information Sciences with the assistance of an Advisory Board, and feedback from consumers and health professionals.

Beyondblue:the national depression initiate

http://www.beyondblue.org.au

Extensive Australian-based site with information for the general public and clinicians on depression and evidence-based treatments.

The Black Dog Institute

http://blackdoginstitute.org.au/

The Black Dog Institute is dedicated to advancing the understanding, diagnosis and management of the depressive disorders.

Post and Antenatal Depression Association Inc (PaNDa)

www.panda.org.au

Provides information to women and their families affected by antenatal and postnatal mood disorders on the causes and symptoms of these disorders, as well as types of treatments and support services are available

The North Queensland Postnatal Distress Support Group (NQPNDG)

www.nqpostnataldistress.com

Information on the causes of Postnatal Depression and recovery patterns of these disorders.

Eating Disorders

Eating Disorders Association (Aust)

http://www.uq.net.au/~zzedianc/

Anxiety Recovery Centre

www.arcvic.com.au

information about anxiety disorders, their management and links

ADAVIC (The Anxiety Disorders Assoc. of Victoria)

www.adavic.org.au

Information about Panic Disorder, Social Phobia, Agrophobia, Generalised Anxiety and Depression and support services

Reconnexion: Treating Panic, Anxiety, Depression and Tranquilliser Dependency

www.tranx.org.au

Information on benzodiazepines (tranquillers and sleeping pills) guidelines on how to use them safely and strategies for sleep and anxiety management.

Social Anxiety Australia

www.socialanxiety.com.au

Information on social anxiety and panic attacks, first-hand accounts from people living with these conditions and links

Anxiety Disorders Alliance

www.ada.mentalhealth.asn.au

Information on anxiety disorders, related resources and support groups

Anxiety Network Australia

www.anxietynetwork.com.au

Information on anxiety disorders, related programs, workshops and courses – as well as stories from people living with these disorders

Clinical Research Unit for Anxiety Disorders (CRUfAD)

www.crufad.org

Information about depression, anxiety and its management

Depression and Mood Disorders Association

http://dmda.mentalhealth.asn.au/supgrp.htm

Mood disorder-related information (eg depression and bipolar disorder), support groups and links

Even Keel

www.evenkeel.org.au

Information on mood disorder-related conditions (e.g. bipolar disorder, schizophrenia, depression, phobias), issues (drug and alcohol use, self-harm) and links

Working Well

www.workingwell.org.au

Supports people in the workplace living with depression

Back from the Brink

www.IamBackFromTheBrink.com

First hand knowledge to consumers, caregivers, and the workplace on how to prevent and overcome depression

Mood GYM

www.moodgym.anu.edu.au

An interactive web-based program that helps people identify problem emotions and develop skills for preventing and managing depression

ARAFMI
(Association for Relatives and Friends of the Mentally Ill)

QLD – www.arafmiqld.org
NSW – www.arafmi.org
SA – www.users.senet.com.au/-panagga/mhrc/
TAS – http://home.iprimus.com.au/rafmi/
VIC – www.arafemi.org.au
WA – www.arafmi.asn.au

Provides information on support services for families and friends of people with mental illness and/or psychiatric disability.

Cyclops ACT

www.cyclopsact.org

Website for young people with a family member who has a mental illness. Find information about illness and disability, about caring for someone and where to get help when things are tough

National Network of Adult and Adolescent Children who have Mentally ill Parents in Victoria (NNAAMI)

www.nnaami.org

This site is run by a group of people who have experienced life with a mentally ill parent - the aim is to provide assistance for each other, via self-help support, discussion and counselling groups

Children of Parents with a Mental Illness (COPMI)

www.copmi.net.au

Contains a database of programs and support services already operating across Australia to support children and families where there is a parent with a mental illness. It also provides access and downloads for a wide variety of resources and support materials and programs, as well as tips provided by its users that have worked for them.

Mensline Australia

www.menslineau.org.au

Information and support for men, especially around family breakdown or separation. This service provides anonymous telephone support, information and referral.

Lifeline

www.lifeline.org.au

Links and a search facility that directs you to your local Lifeline centre

Mental Health Associations/Foundation

NSW – www.mentalhealth.asn.au
NT – www.teamhealth.asn.au
SA – www.users.senet.com.au/-panangga/mhrc
QLD – www.mentalhealth.org.au
VIC – www.mentalhealthvic.org.au
WA – www.waamh.org.au

Information on mental health, research, programs, services and links

Mental Illness Fellowship of Australia

www.schizophrenia.org.au

Information about mental illness, related projects, programs and services in which the organization is involved

SA Drought Link

www.service.sa.gov.au/drought.asp

Drought related information and links, including information on dealing with stress and tough times

Suicide Prevention

Lifeline

www.lifeline.org.au

Links and a search facility that directs you to your local Lifeline centre

Suicide Helpline

www.suicidehelpline.org.au

Information on why a person becomes suicidal, helping someone who is suicidal, what to do in an emergency and how to cope with a death by suicide

Suicide Prevention Australia – SPA

www.suicidepreventionaust.org

Links and referrals to suicide prevention related help lines and services throughout Australia

Telephone Assistance

Suicide Prevention - Suicide Hot Lines

Lifeline 13 11 14

The Salvation Army has a 24-hour Care Line: 1300 36 36 22

Suicide Prevention Crisis Line: (02) 9311 2000

NSW Suicide Prevention & Crisis Intervention 1300 363 622

Crisis Line Northern Territory 1800 019 116

Queensland Crisis Counselling Service 1300 363 622
(same number as NSW and Salvos)

South Australia Mental Health Assessment & Crisis Intervention Service
13 14 65

Tasmania - Samaritans Lifelink - Country 1300 364 566

Tasmania Samaritans Lifelink - metropolitan (03) 6331 3355

Victoria Suicide Help Line 1300 651 251

Western Australia Samaritans Suicide Emergency Service -
Country 1800 198 313

Western Australia Emergency Service - metropolitan 08 9381 5555

ACT Crisis Assessment & Treatment Team 1800 629 354

Telephone Assistance

Kids Help Line – 1800 551 800

Telephone and online counselling for children and young people

Beyond Blue Info Line – 1300 22 4636

Information about depression and anxiety, available treatments and where to get help.

Black Dog Institute

Prince of Wales Hospital has specialised clinics which operate 9 to 5 Monday to Friday.

Bipolar Disorders & Depression Clinic – (02) 9382 2991

Perinatal Clinic – (02) 9382 6665

Mental Health Association NSW – 1300 794 991

Anxiety Disorders Support & Information – 1300 794 992

Mental Health Foundation ACT – 1800 629 354

Mental Health Foundation of Australia (Victoria) – (03) 9427 1294

Mental Health Association (Queensland) – (07) 3271 5544

TEAM Health (Northern Territory) – 1300 780 081 or (08) 8948 4399

Western Australia Association for Mental Health – (08) 9420 7277

Mental Health Coalition of SA Inc. – (08) 8212 8873

Mental Health Foundation of Australia (Victoria) (03) 9427 0406

Drought Link Hotline – 180 2020

To link rural people affected by the drought with services and information

Drought Link Support Worker – 1800 619 532

Personal, family and support line – 24 hours, 7 days a week)

Advice and information about coping with distress and hardship

"Just Ask" National Rural Mental Health Information Service – 1300 13 11 14

An information and referral service for anyone who seeks mental health information, including local services, books, web sites and self-help information such as a "Toolkit for getting through the drought".

Mensline Australia – 1300 78 99 78

A dedicated service for men with relationship and family concerns, staffed by professional counsellors experienced in men's issues. Includes services focussed on Indigenous men, men from Vietnamese and Arabic speaking communities and young men aged 18 to 25 years. A local call 24 hours a day, 7 days a week

GROW Groups

GROW – National Support Office: (07) 3397 7629

GROW – ACT (02) 6295 7791	GROW - NSW (02) 9633 1800
GROW – NT (08) 8985 4799	GROW – QLD (07) 3394 4344
GROW – SA (08) 8244 9299	GROW – TAS (03) 6223 6284
GROW – VIC (03) 9528 2977	GROW – WA (08) 9315 1666

Helpful Books

Learned Optimism – Optimism is essential for a good and suc-cessful life, **Martin Seligman**

What you can change and what you can't change – the complete guide to successful self-improvement

Radical Forgiveness, **Colin Tipping**

Stop Struggling – the how-to of personal change, **Rita Spencer**

The Drama of the Gifted Child – The search for the true self, **Alice Miller**

Potatoes not Prozac, **Kathleen DesMaisons**

Learning to Love Yourself, **Sharon Wegscheider-Cruse**

The Anger Workbook, **Lorraine Bilodeau**

Love is Letting Go of Fear, **Gerald G Jampolsky**

Out of Darkness into the Light – a journey of inner healing, **Gerald G Jampolsky**

Stress Busters, **Amanda Gore**

Being Happy – A Handbook to Greater Confidence and Security, **Andrew Matthews**

Anxiety Disorders Support and Information

Support Groups – 1300 794 992

Self Help Groups – (02) 9339 6093

SANE Australia Help line – 1800 18 SANE or
(03) 9682 5933

Multicultural Mental Health Australia – (02) 9840 3333

Post and Ante Natal Depression Association

Support: 1300 726 306

Maternal & Child Health Line: 132 229

Parentline: 132 289

Post and Ante Natal Depression Support Groups

ACT – (02) 6232 6538
Victoria – (03) 9428 4600
WA – (08) 9340 1622
North Qld – (07) 4728 1911
Tasmania – (03) 6266 3497
NT – (08) 8973 6188
SA – 1800 182 098

References

The Amino Revolution, Dr Robert Erdman & Meiron Jones

H. Schulz & M Jobert, Effects of Hypericum extract on the Sleep EEG in Older Volunteers. J. Geriatric Psychiatry Neurol. 1994, Suppl. S39–S43

B Staffeldt. et al., Pharmacokinetics of Hypericin after oral intake of the hypericum perforatum extract LI 160 in healthy volunteers, J Geriatric Psychiatry Neurol. 1994; suppl 1, S 47–S53

Suzuki O et al, Inhibition of monoamone oxidase by hypericum. Planta Med 1984;3;272–274

Inhibition of MAO & COMT by Hypericum Extracts & Hypericin, J. Geriatric Psychiatry Neurol. 1994; 7, suppl 1, S54–S56

Linde K, et al. St John's wort for major depression. Cochrane Database of Systematic Reviews 2008(4): CD00448, doi:10.1002/14651858.CD000448. PUB3.

Hall RCW, Joffe JR. "Hypomagnesemia; physical and psychiatric symptoms" JAMA 224 (13); 1749–51, 1973

Benton D, Cook R. "The Impact of selenium supplementation on mood" Biol. Psychiatry 29(11); 1092–8, 1991

Maes M, et al, "Hypozincemia in Depression" J. Affective Disorders 31(2); 135–40, 1994

Werbach MR, Nutritional Influences on Mental Illness, Tarzana, California, Third Line Press Inc. 1991

Evans, K. Brain food: the natural cure for depression. Alternative Medicine Magazine 2005 March: 73–75, 97, 100–103. Des Jarlais, G. Alternatives to Prozac. Alternative Medicine Magazine 2005 March: 76. Birdsall, TC. 5-Hydroxytryptophan: a clinically-effective serotonin precursor. Alternative Medicine Review 1998 Aug; 3(4):271–80. Meyers, S. Use of neurotransmitter precursors for treatment of depression. Alternative Medicine Review 2000 Feb; 5(1):64–71.

L- Tryptophan in treatment of restless legs. American Journal Psychiatry 143(4):554–5, 1986

Dopamine -Stice E, et al, Relationship between obesity and blunted striatal response to food, Science 2008; 322:449–452

Singh A, Berk M. Acute management of bipolar disorders, Australian Prescriber 2008;31:73–76

Keks N, Hope J. Treatment-resistant depression. Medical Observer 15 August 2008.

Scientists test 'happy' gene February 26, 2009 news.com

Wilson CJ et al. Cytokines and Cognition – The case for a head to toe inflammatory paradigm. Geriatric Bioscience 2002 50;12:2049

Stewart JW et al. Low B6 levels in depressed outpatients. Biol Psychiat 1984;19(4):613–616

Alpert JE et al. Nutrition and Depression: the role of folate. Nutr Rev 1997;55(5):145–9

Zucker DK et al. B12 deficiency and psychiatric disorders: Case report and literature review. Biol Psychiat 1981;16:197–205

Seidman SN. Testosterone deficiency and mood in ageing men: pathogenic and therapeutic interactions. World J Biol Psychiatry 2003 Jan;4(1):14–20

Meyers, S. Use of neurotransmitter precursors for treatment of depression. Alternative Medicine Review 5(1):64–71, 2000

***http://articles.mercola.com/sites/articles/archive/2009/01/22/
fascinating-facts-you-never-knew-about-the-human-brain.aspx***

Glossary

Autonomic nervous system

Forms part of the peripheral nervous system and controls organs of the body such as the intestines, heart and stomach. In most cases the autonomic nervous system controls unconscious body functions.

Central nervous system

Part of the nervous system comprising of the brain and spinal cord.

Frontal lobes

The part of the brain that governs our personality and emotions. The frontal lobes are involved in decision making, motor function, memory, language, impulse control and social behaviour. They are located at the front of the brain.

Grey matter

The part of the central nervous system that consists of nerve cell bodies. In contrast, white matter consists of nerve fibres.

Limbic system

Consists of a number of components of the brain including the hypothalamus, the hippocampus, the amygdala and others. It largely controls our emotional life and memories.

Melatonin

A hormone produced by the pinel gland of the brain that governs the body's sleep-wake cycle. Melatonin can be prescribed by a doctor to aid the treatment of insomnia or jet lag.

Monoamine oxidase inhibitor

A class of antidepressant drugs that work by preventing the breakdown of monoamine neurotransmitters, primarily noradrenalin and dopamine.

Neurone

A nerve cell.

Neurotransmitter

Chemicals that enable nerve cells to communicate with each other.

Obsessive compulsive disorder

Is a type of anxiety disorder involving obsession (repeated unwanted thoughts that produce anxiety) and compulsions (repetitive rituals done in an attempt to relieve the anxiety).

Psychosis

People with psychosis are not able to distinguish what is real from what is imagined. They typically experience hallucinations, delusions and confused thinking. Psychosis may be part of schizophrenia or just be a one off episode.

Selective Serotonin Reuptake Inhibitors (SSRIs)

A class of antidepressant drugs that allow more serotonin to be available to nerve cells.

Tricyclic antidepressant

A class of antidepressant drugs that allow more serotonin and noradrenalin to be available to nerve cells.

White matter

See grey matter.